Essential Keys to Your Newborn's Sleep

Help Your Newborn Sleep Better Now and Throughout the First Year

Nicole Johnson
Founder of The Baby Sleep Site®

Miriam Chickering
RN, BSN, IBCLC

Copyright Notice:
Copyright © The Baby Sleep Site®, 2013, All rights reserved.
No part of this publication may be reproduced or transmitted in any form or by any means, mechanical or electronic, including photocopying and recording, or by any information storage and retrieval system, without permission in writing from the publisher.

Legal Notice:
While all attempts have been made to verify information provided in this publication, The Baby Sleep Site® does not assume any responsibility for errors, omissions, or contrary interpretation of the subject matter herein.

While The Baby Sleep Site® publishes what we consider to be safe tips and suggestions, all The Baby Sleep Site® content is made available on an as-is basis, with no warrantees expressed or implied. As such, readers use any advice at their own risk. This publication is not intended for use as a source of medical advice.

The Purchaser or Reader of this publication assumes responsibility for the use of these materials and information. The Author assumes no responsibility or liability whatsoever on the behalf of any Purchaser or Reader of these materials.

ISBN-13: 978-1493562442
ISBN-10: 1493562444

CONTENTS

Introduction	1
Essential Key #1: Feeding and Sleep	3
Hunger Cues	3
Newborn Feeding and Sleep Schedules	4
Breastfeeding Your Newborn	5
Bottle Feeding Your Newborn	8
Feeding Tips	10
Essential Key #2: Communication and Sleep	17
Bonding with Your Newborn	19
How to Soothe Your Newborn	21
Swaddling	23
Colic and Crying	25
"Baby Talk"	33
Essential Key #3: Schedules and Sleep	37
Day/Night Confusion	40
Managing Twins and Multiples	42
Your Baby's Changing Sleep Patterns	44
Foundation for Healthy Sleep Habits	45
Gentle Methods to Shift Sleep	46
Establishing Fixed Points	48
Sample Daily Routines	51
Managing Older Children When You Have a Newborn	62

Essential Key #4: Routines and Sleep	67
Approaches to Routine	67
Managing Odd Days, Illnesses and Growth Spurts	70
Helping Your Baby Fall Asleep	73
Developing Healthy Sleep Habits	79
Conclusion	83
About the Authors	85
About The Baby Sleep Site®	87
Additional Support and Resources	89
Ordering Additional Copies	91

INTRODUCTION

As the mom or dad of a newborn, you've likely already discovered that being a parent is a truly unique experience. Nothing else is as exciting and confusing and exhausting and inspiring as being the mom or dad of a precious child! Understandably, nothing can truly prepare someone for becoming a parent.

One of the things that many parents of newborns feel quite unprepared for is sleep (or, rather, the lack of sleep!). Yes, people may have warned you that having a newborn at home is exhausting, but hearing about it is very different than experiencing it first-hand!

As you've no doubt seen for yourself (or will see, if you have a little one on the way), your newborn's sleeping habits and patterns are very different from yours. And that may make it hard for you to understand them. You may be asking yourself questions like,

- "How much sleep does my baby actually need? Is she getting enough?"
- "Why is my baby sleeping so much during the day, and so little at night?"
- "When should my baby be sleeping, and when should he be eating?"
- "Why do my baby's sleeping patterns seem to change from day to day?"

- "My baby seems so tired; why won't she stop crying and fall asleep?"
- "Why does my baby fall asleep in my arms, or in his swing, but not in his crib?"

Not to worry; by the time you've finished reading this e-book, you'll be able to answer all of these questions (and more!), and you'll have a much better understanding of why your newborn sleeps the way he does, and what you can do to help him sleep well.

This book is based on one very simple, straightforward principle, a principle that makes newborn sleep much easier to understand: **everything about a newborn is connected.** How well your baby sleeps depends on a number of other factors, including her feeding patterns, her daily routines, and your ability to respond to her subtle signals about her needs. You'll learn how to "set the stage" for sleep. Setting the stage for sleep is the best way to guide your newborn into healthy sleep habits because you'll learn how to live in harmony with her by meeting and anticipating her needs through listening to her cues, providing an environment that enhances her growth, guiding her through difficult situations, and forming strong bonds through intimate moments spent together.

In this book, Nicole Johnson, the Founder of The Baby Sleep Site®, and Miriam Chickering, an RN, and a Sleep and Board Certified Lactation Consultant, will share what they've learned through personal and professional experience. They will talk about your baby's basic needs, and how they relate to his sleep. You will learn how to lay the foundation for healthy sleep habits, and how to create routines that will promote better, more predictable sleep for your baby. You will learn what his body language and cues mean, as well as how to meet (and even anticipate) his needs. Before you know it, you'll be an expert on your baby, and you'll achieve better sleep for your entire family!

Let's get started!

ESSENTIAL KEY #1: FEEDING AND SLEEP

Hunger Cues

In the newborn stage, feeding drives sleep. This might seem obvious, but it's worth repeating: a hungry baby can't sleep well. In this way, and for this reason, feeding and sleep are closely connected in the newborn stage.

It can sometimes be difficult to tell when a newborn needs to eat. They can't exactly ask for a feeding, after all! But in one sense, your newborn can tell you she is hungry -- she can tell you using hunger cues. Common newborn hunger cues include:

- opening mouth and/or smacking lips
- sucking (on fingers, toes, clothing, lips, etc.)
- "rooting" (moving head around, seeking nipple with mouth)
- fussing or crying

Remember, crying is the last hunger cue your baby will display; your baby will cue with rooting or sucking in the early stages of hunger. So be on the lookout for those early hunger cues, and offer feeds accordingly.

Planning Around Hunger Cues

You do not always have to wait for hunger cues to offer a feed. For example, if you are leaving the house for a few hours, offer a feeding just before you leave, even if it isn't technically "time" for a feed, and even if your baby isn't cueing for a feed yet. Your baby will likely still eat, and then perhaps nap while you are out and about. Or, let's say you have a fitness class at 9:00 a.m. on Thursdays. Offer a feeding at 8:30; this will get you through your class without having to stop and feed.

This same principle applies to sleep, too. Offer a feeding right before bedtime, even if your baby doesn't seem hungry. This can help extend the time between nighttime feedings.

Newborn Feeding and Sleep Schedules

Some parents (especially those who are schedule-oriented themselves) are eager to help their babies establish predictable eating and sleeping schedules right from the beginning. However, most babies are not ready for a set schedule in the first few months of life. The hormones that influence sleep in adults do not have the exact same effects on a newborn, and they need very different sleep and wake cycles for optimal development. If their brains were to follow the same sleep patterns as adults, they would have severe developmental issues; in fact, some research seems to show newborns that experience long and deep sleep states are at a higher risk for SIDS. In order for newborns to develop into healthy babies and toddlers, they need frequent feedings and shorter sleep cycles. Once a baby's gut and internal clocks have developed, they'll begin to display patterns similar to older babies and toddlers. It isn't that newborns need to "normalize" because what they are doing is, in fact, normal and healthy; it's just that they need time to develop. It's pretty amazing that with all of these big jobs to do, some newborns will be sleeping a four (or more) hour stretch by the time they are a few weeks old!

Therefore, it is important to take recommendations about feeding and sleeping times and amounts as exactly that - recommendations, and not exact requirements. As your baby grows, she will likely become more predictable in her eating and sleeping patterns; at that point, she may be ready for more fixed points in her daily schedule. During the newborn stage, however, it is best for everyone to keep feeding and sleeping times flexible. Keep in mind that no one knows your baby like you do, so don't be afraid to listen to your baby and your instincts.

Breastfeeding Your Newborn

Breastfeeding During the First Few Weeks

If you would like your baby to be exclusively breastfed, then mom's focus during the first few weeks of baby's life should be on establishing the breastfeeding relationship, and milk supply. During those initial weeks, it is recommended that babies breastfeed on demand, and be encouraged to suckle at the breast for comfort. Don't spend time looking at the clock; rather, allow your baby to nurse for as long as he seems interested. This will help you establish your milk supply, and it will help your baby learn the mechanics of latching on and suckling at the breast.

Miriam shares:

Before I was a Lactation Consultant, one healthcare provider encouraged me to nurse for only 10 minutes at a time. It wasn't until much later that I learned that newborns can take a long time to complete a feed, and nursing in the early days isn't always about intake. It's just as much about building a supply, and giving your body the hormone signals it needs to make more milk and lay the foundation for a long term milk supply. With my next baby, I learned to encourage my baby to breastfeed for as long as he wanted in the early days; breastfeeding went smoothly, and my baby was happier and more content with more time at the breast.

Creating a Flexible Schedule for Breastfeeding and Sleep

Once nursing is well-established (usually in the first month after birth), you can begin to think about working toward a loosely-organized, flexible feeding and sleep schedule. As you do, keep the following points in mind:

- Most newborns will nurse 10-12 (or more) times in 24 hours.
- Newborns should not go more than 3-4 hours without a feeding, and breastfeeding newborns should be offered a feeding every 2-3 hours during the day.

Typical feedings will last 20-45 minutes (although, they can take as long as an hour in those early weeks!). However, if feedings routinely last an hour or more, there may be a problem with the latch or the amount of milk going to the baby, so check with your baby's health care provider. Be sure to listen to your baby and your body. Breastfeeding should be comfortable, and if it isn't, make sure you see a lactation consultant right away. Pain may mean that your nipples are being damaged or your baby is getting milk too quickly or not getting enough milk. Sometimes leaning back like you would in a recliner while feeding your baby will help her take a bigger mouthful of breast. Don't be afraid to try something new and move around until you and your baby find a comfortable position.

Occasionally, you may notice that your newborn nurses for 15-20 minutes then falls asleep for 20 minutes, followed by a second nursing session. It may feel like he doesn't need this second session, but this is when your baby will get milk with a higher fat content. It's kind of like the coffee break after Thanksgiving dinner – the pause between the main meal and dessert! After this feeding, it is very common for babies to sleep an hour or more.

Newborns often "cluster feed," which simply means they will nurse frequently for a period of time. Cluster feeding is normal for newborns. During cluster feeds, your baby will nurse almost constantly for a few hours and then sleep for several hours straight. Breastfeeding newborns need about 16 hours of total sleep per day. That **sleep will happen in 1-4 hour "chunks"**, with feedings between each period of sleep.

Safety Tip: Babies should have regained their birth weight within 10 days of birth, and then gain ¾ of an ounce to one ounce per day. If you have any concerns about your baby's growth, sleep patterns, or breastfeeding behavior, take him to his doctor or your lactation consultant. **A baby's weight gain is the best indicator of healthy growth.**

All Babies are Different, and So Are All Moms!

As you work to establish a good breastfeeding routine with your baby, remember that every baby is different. What works for other babies might not work for yours. So if your baby doesn't follow these guidelines perfectly, try not to worry (which is easier said than done when you're a new parent!).

Remember, too, that just as every baby is different, every mom is different! This is especially true when it comes to breastfeeding. One mom's breast milk supply and storage capacity, or how much milk she can store in her breasts at one time, will be very different than another mom's.

Think of your breasts like two measuring cups. Each woman has a different sized set of measuring cups (Note: this has nothing to do with the size of your breasts, but internal milk storage capacity – small breasts can have large milk capacity!). In fact, some women find that each breast is a different size! Most women find when they pump that one breast will supply more milk than the other. For instance, one breast may provide 3 ounces and the other breast may provide 4 ounces.

Some moms may want to have an idea of how much their baby takes at a feeding. You can pump your breasts when they feel full (using a high-quality breast pump) to find out how much milk your breasts can store at one time. Usually, you will get the most milk before the first nursing of the day. You can pump two hours or so before your baby's first feeding. This will allow your breasts time to make more milk for your baby, if you prefer not to give her the pumped breast milk from a bottle. (Tip: Do not routinely offer a bottle to your baby until the breastfeeding relationship is established, which usually happens around 3-4 weeks old. This will help your baby avoid nipple confusion.) Some moms get an idea of their storage capacity by pumping; however, be aware that your baby will likely be able to draw more milk out of your breast than the pump will, and some moms don't respond well to a pump. You might use hand expression of breast milk as an alternative or in addition to a pump. If you don't feel the pump is helpful for determining your storage capacity, you may choose to have your baby weighed before the feeding, between breasts (if he is taking both breasts), and after the feeding. This will also give you a very good idea of your storage capacity, especially if you do it during the first feeding of the day, as that is often one of the larger feedings of the day.

A woman with large "cups" may be able to go longer between feedings, while a woman with smaller "cups" may have to nurse more frequently, since her baby doesn't consume as much milk during each feeding. What's more, a woman with a smaller storage capacity will need to nurse more frequently to empty her breasts and make room for more breast milk, because empty breasts make milk more quickly than full breasts.

Bottle Feeding Your Newborn

Choosing the Right Bottle and Nipple

The question of which bottle or nipple is right for your baby depends entirely on preference -- both yours and your newborn's! So at first, you may need to use a "trial and error" approach to finding the right bottle and nipple.

Here are some tips that may help you decide which bottles and nipples to start with:

- If you use a plastic bottle, be sure that it's BPA-free.
- Begin with smaller-sized bottles (4 or 6 ounce); these are perfect for the amount of breast milk or formula your newborn will need at the start. As your baby grows, you can transition to larger-sized bottles.
- If you'll be exclusively formula feeding, you'll need plenty of bottles. Aim for having 10-12.
- There are many different shapes of bottle nipples available. Some nipples are designed to mimic the shape and feel of mom's breast; if you want to switch back and forth between breast and bottle feeding, these may be a good option.
- Newborns should begin with the smallest-sized nipples (usually known as "stage 1" nipples) and graduate to larger sizes as they get older. This will ensure that the flow of formula is not too fast for your newborn. If you are breastfeeding, you may never graduate to faster flow nipples, so you can mimic the breast. Some babies begin to get frustrated at the breast, if the milk does not flow as quickly as a Stage 2 or 3 nipple, for example.

Nicole shares:

My sons struggled to take the bottle, at first, but once they did, we never increased the nipple sizes in order to mimic my breasts. In the end, they both struggled to give up bottles and one even more so than breastfeeding!

Choosing the Right Formula

Milk-based formulas are the most common types of infant formulas available, and many babies do well with these. For babies with milk allergies, soy-based formulas are available. (Note: Do not switch to a soy-based formula unless directed by your doctor.) If your baby has problems digesting milk and soy formulas, protein hydrolysate formula is available. Protein hydrolysate formula contains proteins that have been partially broken down, making them easier for baby to digest.

When it comes to brands of formula, there are many to choose from -- and that can be overwhelming! It may be helpful for you to know that, from a nutritional standpoint, these formulas are essentially the same. In the United States, the FDA (Food and Drug Administration) carefully regulates infant formula, and all formula manufacturers must follow a strict set of standards. The same is true in some other countries as well. So name-brand formulas aren't necessarily "better" than generic formulas. Therefore, the brand of formula you choose can be based on your baby's preferences (and your own). You might research the number of recalls a particular brand has had before choosing. Some babies are sensitive to a change between brands, so you may want to talk with your doctor before switching. Ultimately, if you have questions or concerns about what type or brand of formula is right for your baby, it is best if you ask your baby's healthcare provider.

Points to Remember When Using Formula

Sleep and feeding schedules are a bit different for formula feeding babies than they are for breastfeeding babies. Babies who drink formula will still need to eat every few hours.

Keep these points in mind as you work towards creating a general, flexible schedule for your baby:

- Newborns will drink about 2-4 ounces of formula per feeding.

- Newborns who are formula-fed will need about 6-8 feedings per day.

- When figuring out how much formula your newborn needs to drink each day, use this simple formula: your baby needs about 2-3 ounces of formula for every pound he weighs. So an 8 pound newborn needs 16-24 ounces of formula per day.

- Formula feedings can be spaced 3-4 hours apart in many cases.

- A typical formula feeding for a newborn will take about 20-30 minutes.

- Formula fed babies may be more likely to "overeat" than breastfed babies. An overly full baby may experience discomfort (gas, vomiting, etc.).

- Formula-feeding newborns need about 16 hours of total sleep per day. That sleep will happen in 1-4 hour "chunks," with feedings happening between each period of sleep.

Feeding Tips

There are many reasons why a mom might choose to supplement breastfeeding with bottle feeding (with a bottle filled with pumped or hand expressed breast milk). Here are a few reasons you may want to consider it:

Supplementing with a Bottle Can Help Mom Get Some Much-Needed Rest

Some moms may feel exhausted in the early weeks after delivery. Offering breast milk in a bottle can help mom get the rest she needs, while ensuring that baby is well-nourished.

Miriam shares that this was the case for a friend of hers:

One of my friends told me that she felt tired and overwhelmed around day 5 after her delivery. She felt that if she didn't get some good sleep, she wouldn't be able to continue breastfeeding. So she pumped one bottle of breast milk. Then, she breastfed her baby right before her (mom's) bedtime. She went to sleep in a quiet part of the house while the baby stayed with her husband. When the baby woke hungry, her daddy gave her the bottle, and my friend was able to get 6 straight hours of sleep! She said it was just the boost she needed to feel recovered from delivery. It wasn't something she did every day, because that could have damaged her milk supply over the long term, but for one or two nights, she found it was a life-saver!

Supplementing Can Help Mom Get Out and About

Moms may find it convenient to pump a bottle that someone else (caregiver, spouse, etc.) can feed the baby when mom leaves the house. Mom may need to pump while she is out, if she'll be gone more than three hours to prevent her breasts from becoming too full, but overall, this can make running errands or meeting up with friends much easier, and can provide mom with a nice break, although some moms may not want a break and may prefer to stay close to home during the first few months – and that's perfectly normal too.

Keep in mind that milk supply isn't fully established until about a month and a half after delivery. Going too long between pumping or feeding can decrease milk supply, and may also lead to your breasts becoming overly full, which can in turn lead to a blocked duct, which may cause infection to set in (called 'mastitis').

Some mothers choose to exclusively pump their breast milk, and this can work very well, if you keep a few things in mind. First, use a high quality breast pump. Second, while pumping, use massage and breast compressions to increase the amount of milk you get with each session and to stimulate your breasts to increase production. Finally, consider using hand expression after each pumping session.

Supplementing Can Help Mom Get Back to Work

Moms who work outside the home but want to continue breastfeeding can do just that, with the help of a high-quality breast pump. (Tip: Many moms are able to get a free pump through their insurance, so be sure to check with yours before you buy.) In preparation for returning to work, moms will want to focus on building a stash of pumped breast milk after delivery. However, it is usually best to begin serious stashing after the first 4-6 weeks. Some moms find that pumping too much before this time causes problems with chronic oversupply of milk.

Working moms may also wish to increase their milk supply (ensuring that they have plenty of breast milk to offer baby). If you're working towards increasing your supply, you can achieve this by pumping for approximately 10 minutes after you finish nursing your baby. You don't have to pump after each feeding, although that will usually lead to a faster increase. Hand-expressing your milk for a few minutes after 5 feedings per day may nearly double your milk supply! Even better, hand expressing for a few minutes after each feeding the first few days after delivery can increase the number of prolactin receptors in your breast, resulting in a larger milk supply for the entire time of breastfeeding.

Once your maternity leave is over and you are back at work, maintain your milk supply by pumping at work during those times that you'd normally be nursing your baby. For instance, if your newborn usually nurses every 2-3 hours during the day, then be sure to pump that frequently while you're at work.

There are some simple techniques that can make a big difference when you need to pump your milk or increase your supply. One such technique is breast massage. Breast massage is done when a mom kneads her breasts for a minute or so before pumping. There is no one right way to do breast massage; however, the massage should be firm and not painful. Breast compressions can be done during pumping to increase flow. Hand expression can be used for a few minutes after pumping; even a drop or two of milk with hand expression is a good start. Laying a warm rice sock across your breasts a few minutes before pumping, or pumping just after a warm shower, can be very helpful as well. Heat, massage, compressions, and hand expression are very powerful tools for increasing the amount of milk you get at each pumping. While it may take some time to get used to all of this hands-on activity, you'll be an expert in no time!

Finally, some working moms may find that "reverse cycling" actually helps them with their pumping and nursing schedules. Reverse cycling occurs when a baby nurses more (and sometimes sleeps less) during the night, while nursing less (and possibly sleeping more) during the day. For many parents, reverse cycling is an understandably frustrating problem that needs to be overcome, and we can help you find a personalized solution with our Newborn Sleep Plans, if you need help. For some working moms, however - especially moms who work part-time and can sleep a bit during the day, or moms who bed-share - reverse cycling actually works well. Reverse cycling allows working moms to nurse often during the night and pump less frequently during the day. What's more, it can be a great way to reconnect with your baby!

Supplementing with Formula

Some moms want (or need) to supplement their breast milk with infant formula. If your baby is currently drinking formula and breastfeeding, and you'd like to work towards exclusively breastfeeding, there is a link to a helpful article with information on how to increase your supply and decrease supplementation a little at a time. on our site which is referenced on the Resource page at the end of this book. Note that while some babies will let you know right away if they're not getting enough to eat (by waking from sleep and crying loudly), others won't. These babies will tend to sleep more when they aren't getting enough to eat, making it hard for parents to spot the problem. For this reason, it's a good idea for your baby to get **regular weight checks** while weaning from supplemental formula.

If you're moving in the other direction, however - if you're exclusively breastfeeding now, and want to work some formula into your feeding routine - it's important to remember that your milk supply isn't fully-established until about a month and a half after delivery. If possible, wait to introduce formula until after that time. If you need to introduce formula before that point, but you'd like to continue partially breastfeeding, you'll probably need to pump or nurse at least once during the night and every 3 hours during the day for the first couple of months, in order to ensure a good supply. Otherwise, you'll tend to have less and less milk over time, until your baby is getting very little breast milk.

Dreamfeeding Your Newborn

One feeding technique that can be really helpful during the newborn stage is the 'dream feed'. Dream feeding works like this: before you go to bed, you wake your baby slightly, feed her, and then put her right back to bed. The idea here is that your baby takes in a full feeding and is then able to sleep for a few more hours -- which means you get to sleep for a few hours!

When they work, dream feeds can be a great tool for parents to use in order to maximize their own sleep. This is especially true during the newborn stage, when babies need to eat so frequently.

Here are a few pointers to help you decide if dream feeding will work for you, and to help you understand how to incorporate it into your baby's evening:

- If your baby is asleep at your bedtime, rouse your baby just enough to offer a feeding - don't wake him up all the way! Of course, you may not be able to rouse your baby enough to get him to take a full feeding; this is okay. If he's really sleepy, encourage him to feed by using skin-to-skin, burping, and breast compressions, but sometimes you'll try all of those things, and he may simply be too sleepy, so be willing to stop when he seems done.
- If your baby doesn't take a full feeding during the dream feed, don't be surprised if he wakes shortly after, for a full feeding.
- If you are breastfeeding, remember that you will need to empty your breasts every few hours, in order to keep up your milk supply.
- Remember that the dream feed is a tool designed to help parents. If you've tried dream feeding for 4 or 5 days, and found that it just isn't working for you and your baby, then don't offer it anymore. The goal of the dream feed is to get your baby's longest sleep stretch to line up with yours, but some babies have difficulty changing that stretch from early evening to late evening and the middle of the night.

Suckling for Comfort

A newborn's suckling reflex is strong, and it's important that newborns be allowed to suckle for comfort. This will help them adjust to life outside the womb as it's very comforting. Some babies have stronger needs to suck than others and all babies are unique in their needs. To satisfy this suckling need, newborns can suckle on a pacifier (or other nipple replacement such as your finger or baby's own hands) or mother's breast, which will be discussed below.

Introducing the Pacifier

Formula-fed babies should use a pacifier during the newborn stage, in order to prevent over-feeding, to reduce the risks associated with SIDS, and to satisfy their suckling reflex. Breastfed babies can benefit from pacifiers, too, although it's generally best to wait until a breastfed baby is one month old before introducing a pacifier, in order to avoid nipple confusion.

Pacifiers provide a great way to soothe and calm babies for a few minutes at a time during diaper and clothing changes, during baths, on short car rides, or anytime she feels stressed and the breast or skin is unavailable. But remember, pacifiers shouldn't be used to delay a feeding. Also keep in mind that while pacifiers can be useful tools, they are not mandatory. So, if your baby does not seem interested in the pacifier, it's nothing to worry about.

Suckling at the Breast

Breastfed newborns need some time to suckle at the breast for comfort. This satisfies your baby's reflexive suckling needs and helps you establish a stable and adequate milk supply. After the first 12-16 weeks have passed, and your baby is moving out of the newborn stage, suckling for comfort becomes more habitual and less reflexive. At this age, infants are able to do the majority of the suckling they need during feeding times.

The exception to this "rule" is those moms who have very large storage capacities and who therefore don't nurse as frequently during the day. These moms may need to provide their babies with additional opportunities to suckle at the breast, as well as providing more time for pacifier use.

Skin to Skin Contact

Skin to skin contact is one of the best ways you can enhance your newborn's feeding times. This is true for both breastfed and bottle fed babies. Practicing skin to skin contact is easy; simply undress your baby down to his diaper, and place him on your bare chest. And remember, this is something both moms and dads can do!

The benefits of skin to skin contact for newborns are numerous. For starters, babies who receive skin to skin contact stabilize much more quickly after birth; they grow better and cry less. Skin to skin contact may also help ensure that newborns feed as frequently as they need to. Even sleepy newborns will usually wake up when they need to eat, if they are placed against mom or dad's skin. But babies who are always wrapped up snugly may sleep through feedings (depending on their temperament and the events surrounding delivery). In this way, skin to skin contact may result in a newborn who regains his birth weight quickly.

Finally, skin to skin contact is also healthy for a newborn's skin and gut. Keep in mind that when babies are born, their bodies don't contain a large amount of the good bacteria that helps keep them healthy. Being exposed to mom and dad's skin helps them develop the healthy bacteria they need to protect against germs and illness.

Having special time with your baby right against your skin is healthy for parents, too! You will have a release of endorphins- which are feel good hormones, and this works to further attachment between mom, dad and baby.

Miriam shares:

I remember how much I enjoyed feeding my first baby, Beka. It was such a relief when feeding time came, because I would take her into my bedroom, and have her all to myself while she breastfed and then we would grab a nap. We used formula too (due to some medical issues), and her dad and grandma enjoyed taking turns with bottle feedings. Those early memories of motherhood and becoming a family of three are incredibly precious.

It's comforting to have the knowledge to ensure your baby is getting all of the nutrition she needs to grow. Feedings and sleep are connected, and now you know how to help her get enough of both.

ESSENTIAL KEY #2: COMMUNICATION & SLEEP

Your newborn obviously can't use words to communicate with you, but she does have a variety of other ways to let you know about her needs -- including her sleep needs. Vocalizations are the noises your newborn makes including cooing, grunting, crying, and other noises. Newborns communicate in three major ways: through vocalizations, through body language, and through reflexive behaviors. In this section, we'll discuss how to interpret your newborn's 'language', so that you can 'hear' what she is saying and perhaps even predict her next need.

Understanding Your Newborn's Vocalizations

Baby noises (including cries) are the most recognizable ways your newborn will communicate with you. The problem is that adults aren't naturally fluent in our babies' language. We don't speak "baby talk!"

Can You Decode Your Baby's Noises?

Conventional wisdom says most parents learn to "decode" their baby's cries, but the truth is, many moms of newborns confess that they have a hard time figuring out what their babies' noises mean. In the early weeks after your baby is born, it can indeed be very hard to tell one cry or vocalization from another.

However, rest assured that over time, you will come to understand your baby's own unique style of vocalization, and you'll be able to better respond. During the newborn phase, however, don't worry if you feel confused by your baby's noises, and don't feel too frustrated if you aren't able to "decode" them right away.

You may not be able to decode all of your newborn's cries at first, but you can certainly take steps to comfort your little one when she's upset. You can use context clues to help you determine what your baby's cries might mean. For instance, if it's been two or three hours since your baby has eaten, it's likely that she's hungry. Or if she's been awake for awhile, she may very well be sleepy and need to nap. Is she drawing her legs up to her belly and grunting? Then she may need to be burped or pass gas.

Priscilla Dunstan & Your Baby's Secret Language

While most of us parents will learn, over time, how to generally interpret our babies' cries, one mom claims that our babies actually speak to us, and that if we can simply learn their "secret language," we can easily meet their needs and reduce crying and sleeplessness. Sound too good to be true? Priscilla Dunstan says it's not.

Australian mom Priscilla Dunstan was born with a rare gift -- she has a photographic memory for sound. This means that Dunstan is able to hear and decode sounds that the rest of us can't. Dunstan says that it wasn't until her son Tom was born in 1998, however, that she realized her gift might actually help her understand her newborn. Dunstan says that she started to hear patterns in Tom's cries, and came to realize that as he vocalized, Tom was trying to tell her what he needed. Dunstan quickly discovered that these sound patterns weren't unique to Tom, however -- she began hearing them in other babies' cries, too. You can find the link to a video of her interview with Oprah on the Resources Page.

Through research and time spent with other babies, Dunstan was able to isolate 5 distinct sounds, or "words", that all babies say. Those words are:

- Neh (meaning "I'm hungry")
- Owh (meaning "I'm sleepy")
- Heh (meaning "I'm uncomfortable")
- Eairh (meaning "I have belly gas")

- Eh (meaning "I need to burp")

Dunstan explains that, in her experience, all babies say these words. Her premise rests on the idea that newborn reflexes lead to specific pre-crying sounds that all newborns make. With careful training and plenty of practice (which she offers on her website, DunstanBaby.com), moms and dads can learn to recognize these words and respond to their babies' needs quickly and correctly.

Bonding With Your Newborn

Few things are stronger than the bond between a parent and a child. For some parents, this bond begins immediately after birth. There's a reason for that -- during labor, mom's body releases lots of the hormone oxytocin, which in turn can cause mom to have strong, overwhelming feelings of love for her baby, as well as the desire to protect her baby.

However, not all parents feel this kind of instant bond with their babies. Many moms feel completely exhausted after delivery. Other moms may begin to experience postpartum depression symptoms just a few days after birth. In these cases, mom may not feel an instant bond with baby -- but that's perfectly okay! Growing close to and 'learning' your baby is a process, after all, and one that can take some time.

'Learning' Your Newborn: The First Step in Bonding

Your newborn will communicate primarily through his body posture, reflexive cues, and cries. But when your baby is first born, you may have a hard time decoding those cries and cues and body language! Don't worry, though; with a little practice and lots of listening, you'll begin to understand what your baby needs and what he's trying to 'tell' you. So, listen to and watch your baby, and before you know it, you'll be the expert on his needs!

Tips for Bonding with Your Newborn

It can be so easy to feel overwhelmed when you have a newborn at home. You likely feel exhausted, thanks to all the nighttime waking. All of your usual responsibilities may feel like more than you can handle, since simply feeding and caring for your newborn is practically its own full-time job! And if you're working on improving your newborn's sleep, it can be easy to over-focus on what is going 'wrong' with your newborn and your schedule. This is understandable, but as much as we want to get sleep "right", the most important thing is that you and your baby feel connected. So while you're working on sleep, be sure to take some extra time to just be together.

Plain old snuggling and cuddling are great ways to bond with your baby. Here are some creative ideas for bonding time:

Take a bath with your newborn baby. Bathing with your baby is a great way to initiate the skin-to-skin contact that is so important for your newborn. That skin-to-skin contact, plus the combination of warm water, can be especially effective at soothing your baby when she is fussy. But remember, safety first! Be sure that someone else is in the bathroom with you, to help you with the baby.

Massage your newborn baby. Massage is an excellent way to calm and soothe your baby, and to strengthen the connection between the two of you. Incorporate some essential oils into your massage routine for an even more soothing massage! (Just be sure to read the article listed on our Resource Page first, for a list of approved essential oils for babies, as well as tips on using essential oils safely). Want to know more about baby massage, or wondering how to begin? There is also an all about infant massage listed on our Resource Page.

Read with and/or sing to your newborn baby. Sure, your baby won't be able to understand the words to your book, or to your song, but that's not the point. Hearing the gentle cadence of your voice, and watching your face, will go a long way in helping your newborn connect with and bond to you.

Learn Baby Sign Language with your baby. Again, in the newborn stage, your baby is too young to actually learn or understand any of the Baby Sign Language signs. But at this stage, that doesn't matter. Simply watching you and listening to your voice is what makes this special (for both of you!) And of course, the added bonus is that as your baby grows, she will likely pick up quickly on the basic signs quickly. This will lay a great foundation for going even farther in learning Baby Sign Language (should you choose to do that).

Take a walk with your baby. If the weather's cooperative, take your baby on a stroll. The fresh air will be great for both of you, and the exercise you get will do wonders for your overall energy! While you walk, don't be shy about talking aloud to your baby -- point out the sights as you pass, name objects for your baby, etc. Getting into this habit now will ensure that as your baby grows, he learns the names for common objects and sights as soon as he's able.

If you have adopted a newborn, skin-to-skin contact and spending time getting to know each other are critically important. Some moms who adopt are able to breastfeed or partially breastfeed. If you're interested, there is an article on our Resources Page about nursing adopted babies or you can find more information about breastfeeding an adopted baby in the book, *The Ultimate Breastfeeding Book of Answers*. You may also want to consider using donated breast milk. We have also included a link to Kellymom.com on our Resource page which is a comprehensive resource about donor breast milk.

Exactly how you bond and connect with your baby isn't important; it's the bonding and connecting that matters. So be sure to take some time, in the midst of all the feedings and night wakings and general busy-ness of those first few months, to simply sit with and enjoy your newborn. That's the first step in creating the kind of strong bonds that will last a lifetime!

How to Soothe Your Newborn

You don't necessarily need to learn the Dunstan Baby Language system (although a number of moms swear that it truly works). Even if you never learn how to translate your baby's "secret language," you can still learn to respond to her cues and comfort your baby when she cries, using some tried-and-true methods that have worked for parents around the world, for generations.

The Karp Method

Dr. Harvey Karp, a pediatrician, became a household name in the United States with the publication of his book, The Happiest Baby on the Block. The basic idea that Karp puts forth in the book is an interesting one: he believes that the first three months of a newborn's life should actually be considered a fourth trimester. He points out that human babies are born quite early, and that loads of brain development take place in the early weeks after birth.

Therefore, says Karp, the best way to soothe a crying newborn is to recreate "womb-like" conditions as best you can. How can moms and dads create a womb-like feel for their newborn? Karp breaks it down into the 5 S's:

Swaddle: Newborns are wrapped up snugly while in the womb, and wrapping our newborns up snugly in a blanket can help recreate that snug, soothing feeling. It's true that many newborns don't like the sensation of being able to flail their arms and legs, and that swaddling seems to provide comfort.

Safety Tip: See section below about safe swaddling techniques and tips.

Side/Stomach Position: It isn't recommended that parents place their babies on their sides or stomachs for sleep. The AAP recommends that the safest way for a baby to sleep is on her back. However, when parents are holding their babies, it can be comforting for the baby to be held on his side or on his stomach. Specifically, parents can hold their babies on their right sides, facing slightly down.

Swinging: When the baby is swaddled and lying face-down in your arms, it's time to start gently swinging the baby back and forth. Note that this isn't supposed to be a fast, jerky swing; it's more of a gentle rocking. This recreates the gentle rocking motion that babies experience in the womb.

Nicole shares:

Of course, my first-born needed to swing fairly hard to be soothed, so all babies are different!

Shushing: In addition to swinging, you can make a loud "shushing" noise close to your baby's ears. This loud, consistent shushing is supposed to mimic the white noise that a baby hears in the womb.

Sucking: The sucking reflex is very strong in a newborn, and very comforting. Babies find comfort at the breast, and formula fed babies can find comfort with a pacifier.

Swaddling

Swaddling is considered an age-old technique for soothing fussy infants -- people around the world have been swaddling their babies for centuries. The act of swaddling is to mimic the womb by wrapping the infant such that he has a 'cocoon' around him (some call it wrapping baby like a burrito). There are correct and incorrect ways to swaddle a newborn, so it's important to do it safely.

8 Tips for Safe Swaddling

Swaddling can be a great way to soothe a fussy newborn; however, it must be done safely. Fortunately, there are several techniques you can use to make swaddling safe for your newborn. Those techniques include:

1. **Don't swaddle too tightly.**

    When you swaddle your baby, you may feel tempted to wrap him up as tightly as possible, so that he'll be less likely to break free. Avoid that impulse. Babies who are wrapped too tightly may not be able to breathe well due to chest constriction, and wrapping their legs too tightly can lead to hip dysplasia and dislocation. A baby's legs should always be able to bend freely in the swaddle. Bottom line: babies should be wrapped snugly, but not tightly, in a light and breathable swaddle blanket or sleep sack.

    You can swaddle your baby using a simple cotton blanket; you can also use specialty swaddling blankets, designed to make the process of swaddling easier. Nicole used the Miracle Blanket with both of her boys.

2. **Keep the swaddle away from the baby's face.**
3. **Stop swaddling once he can roll.**
4. **Place him on his back to sleep.**
5. **If you intend to swaddle your baby during sleep, begin at birth, don't begin after he is several months old.**
6. **Don't swaddle when he has a fever or is ill.**
7. **Choose a good arm/hand position.**

Historically, parents have swaddled babies with their arms by their sides. Recently, however, there's been a push to swaddle babies with their hands by their faces. Supporters of this technique point out that it allows babies to self-soothe, by sucking on their fingers. Babies with their hands near their faces are also more likely to cue for a feeding, while babies wrapped with their hands by their sides are more likely to sleep through a feeding. This can have big implications for some breastfed babies, because some babies may sleep through needed feedings. It may be best to swaddle with hands at the sides solely for soothing purposes, instead of as a routine measure. They also point out that wrapping with one or both hands near the face gives baby a bit more mobility, which means that if your baby does accidentally roll over while swaddled, she may be able to do something about it.

However, not everyone agrees. In a phone interview with Nicole, Dr. Karp explained that he still advocates for swaddling with arms by the sides. He shared that after the first few weeks of a baby's life, his arms begin to relax, and it's more comfortable for most babies to have hands by the sides. He also pointed out that if babies' hands are by their faces, they're less likely to soothe themselves and more likely to hit or scratch themselves in the face (which is decidedly un-soothing!) He also pointed out that a baby who's swaddled with hands by face is far more likely to break free of the swaddle, and that means loose blankets in the crib, which is a safety concern.

All babies are different, so listen to your baby's cues about what is most comfortable for her. If you do swaddle with arms by sides, be sure to leave a little flexion in the elbows — your baby's arms shouldn't be rigidly straight. If you swaddle with hands by face, be aware that you may need to check on baby regularly, to be sure she hasn't loosened her blanket or broken free of the swaddle.

8. Supervising your baby. To be completely safe, you should supervise your baby while he's swaddled. That way, if the blankets come loose, or if he rolls over, you're there to intervene. Many families of newborns tend to room-share for closer monitoring during sleep. If you're practicing safe swaddling techniques (using light cotton blankets, swaddling snugly but not tightly, etc.), you greatly reduce the risk that anything dangerous can happen to your baby while he's swaddled.

However, to be extra cautious, if you want to swaddle your baby for prolonged periods of time at night, you could invest in a movement monitor, like the Snuza™. A movement monitor does just what the name says — it monitors your baby's movements. If your baby is completely still for too long, an alarm should sound, letting you know about it. Movement monitors are designed to alert parents (or daycare staffers) to situations in which a baby might not be breathing. Movement monitors can provide parents extra peace of mind, but they are not approved medical devices for monitoring breathing or oxygen levels like monitors that you might see in a NICU. Under-the-mattress monitors (like the Angel Care Monitor) are also available; they're designed to fit under your baby's crib sheets, as opposed to clipping onto your baby's pajamas.

For a video demonstration of safe swaddling techniques, please watch the video listed on our Resources Page.

Colic and Crying

Why Do Newborns Cry?

The list of reasons why your newborn baby may cry is a long one. Newborns cry because:

- they're hungry.
- they're sleepy.
- their diaper is wet or dirty.
- they're uncomfortable.
- they're over-stimulated.
- they're gassy.
- they're too hot (or too cold).
- they want to be held.

Why Do Babies Cry When They're Tired?

Some of these reasons are easy to understand – when early cues are missed, most hungry babies will obviously cry for food (however, personalized consultations tell us that there are a rare few who don't), and an uncomfortable baby will cry until she's made comfortable again. But many parents struggle to understand why their newborns cry when they're tired. Why wouldn't a tired newborn simply fall asleep?

If only it were that easy! The truth is, newborns become overly-tired very quickly. And once a newborn is overtired, it becomes difficult for her wind down and fall asleep. Your newborn will become fussy when she starts feeling sleepy, but very quickly, her fussiness will escalate into full crying and then screaming as she becomes overly-exhausted. By that point, it can be impossible for your newborn to fall asleep without first being soothed by you. The great news, however, is that a close cuddle, or a few minutes rocking or suckling, will often be enough to soothe your baby to sleep.

We are going to discuss some great methods to prevent and decrease crying, and with this knowledge, you will be able to dramatically reduce the amount your baby cries. Even so, there will be times you will quickly attend to your baby and address every conceivable need (hunger, discomfort, exhaustion, loneliness, etc.), and your baby will still cry; that's okay. Once you have done everything you can to soothe your baby and your baby is still crying, it's great to remind yourself of this fact: **A crying baby does not equal bad parents.**

Some newborns cry so often, and so inconsolably, that it seems to go beyond the standards of normal. These newborns will sometimes cry for hours on end, and their parents' comforting measures seem to be ineffective. Crying like this is typically called colic (even when it isn't true colic). Excessive crying is very upsetting to parents and babies. Sometimes, healthcare professionals and parents are able to find a specific cause. Some of the most common causes of excessive crying are the following:

- **Dairy Allergy** - Dairy allergies stem from cow's milk based formula or dairy in mom's diet, if she's breast feeding. If dairy is the culprit, removing it from moms and baby's diet for 3-4 days should result in some improvement of symptoms, although things may continue to improve over the next two weeks.

- **Reflux** – This is very common in babies and doesn't need treatment unless it becomes a problem. Doctors can treat this with medication, but small frequent feedings and keeping baby upright for 15-30 minutes after a feeding can help.

- **Oversupply** – Some breastfed babies can become excessively fussy when mom has too much breast milk. Sometimes this can be difficult to spot since these babies don't get enough of the fatty milk and constantly want to go to the breast. Since the babies are constantly going to the breast, mom may think she doesn't have enough milk. If you are breastfeeding and your baby is excessively fussy, see an IBCLC (independent board certified lactation consultant).

- **Tongue Tie** – Both breast and bottle feeding babies tend to cry more when they can't feed properly due to tongue tie. Both obvious tongue ties and posterior tongue ties can cause problems. A lactation consultant can help you evaluate your baby for tongue tie, and a doctor or pediatric dentist can correct a tongue tie.

- **Formula Feeding** – Some babies who receive formula can have inflamed guts. Sometimes, switching to a special formula, switching to human donor milk from a milk bank, or giving probiotics (approved by the doctor) can help.

- **Problems with the Spine or Muscles** – Some families report that a trip to a chiropractor, physical therapist, or cranial-sacral therapist really helped decrease their baby's crying. You may want to check with your primary care physician before seeing a specialist for more information.

- **Temperament and Maturity** – Once other things have been ruled out, we should consider temperament and maturity. Some babies simply have a more difficult time adjusting to the outside world. Transitioning between states is very difficult to them. The absolute best way to help these babies is by increasing the contact they have with a caregiver who can help them regulate their awake and sleep states. These babies need soothing, consistent routines, loving interaction, and LOTS and LOTS of physical contact, including skin to skin contact (see page 16).

What is Colic?

The term colic refers to extended periods of crying -- three or more hours -- that happen three or more times per week, during the first few months of life. Colic happens most often in the late afternoon and evening (although it can happen any time of the day). It's estimated that about 20% of newborns suffer through colic -- and their parents suffer with them!

Miriam shares:

Hannah, my niece, had colic. She cried from 9 pm to 12 am every night for months. She cried with less intensity when my sister offered the breast, skin to skin, or when she was swaddled and 'Karped' with the five 'S', but she still cried. If she was put down in her crib, the crying would escalate to a scream; the soothing helped, but didn't fix the crying. Those were some difficult nights to get through, but it helped to know that the colicky crying would end, and it did. It stopped when she was about 14 weeks old, and now she is a very pleasant and healthy toddler.

Unfortunately, there's no one known cause of colic. People have long thought that colic must be caused by digestive problems, like gas and reflux; however, researchers haven't been able to define a single cause of colic, despite numerous studies. The good news is that there are things you can do to decrease crying even if your baby does have colic. The comfort measures you use with your baby may not put a stop to the crying, but experts estimate that comfort measures reduce colic crying by 50%.

Newborns Need Help Regulating Their Responses

The term 'colic' has long been applied to any baby who cries loudly and inconsolably for long periods of time. The problem with this, however, is that saying, "Your baby must have colic" implies that there's something wrong with the crying baby, and that his crying is unnatural or abnormal. In reality, doctors and medical researchers now believe that all babies go through a time when they are not very good at regulating their responses to the outside world with all its new sensations. Sometimes, this results in crying. These doctors and researchers refer to colic as The Period of Purple

Crying (www.purplecrying.info). The Period of Purple Crying begins around 2 weeks of age, and it lasts until 3-4 months of age. During this window of time, some babies will go through 'colicky' crying spells.

It should be noted that the world purple here doesn't refer to the actual color purple (as in "My baby cries until he turns purple!"). Rather, it's used as an acronym:

P - Peak of Crying. The length of time your baby spends crying will increase each week, peaking sometime in month 2, and then decreasing during month 3 or 4.

U - Unexpected. Your baby's crying will come and go, start and stop -- and you won't know why.

R - Resists Soothing. No matter what you do to soothe her, your baby will cry.

P - Pain-like Face. Your baby may grimace as if he's in pain when he's crying. While this is understandably alarming to parents, rest assured that if you've tried to make your baby comfortable and he's still crying, then he's probably not in actual pain. (Although if this is a new type of crying, especially a high pitched cry, you should have him evaluated by his health care provider.)

L - Long-lasting. Crying may last for hours each day.

E - Evening. Your baby is more likely to cry inconsolably during the late afternoon and evening.

Babies, from about 2 weeks until about 3-4 months, go through this Period of Purple Crying. Young brains are developing, and during all of these huge changes, newborns are being exposed to a wonderful and overwhelming new world. For many babies, the crying isn't excessive, and parents are able to manage it well by responding quickly to cues and anticipating needs. For others, however, the crying is intense and exhausting even when they receive a great deal of responsive parenting. The reason why some babies pass through this phase peacefully and others don't probably has a lot do to with each baby's temperament. Some babies are very intense and/or perceptive, and these babies are more likely to cry inconsolably than relaxed babies are. (See link on the Resources Page for more information about baby temperaments and sleep.)

Speaking of intense and perceptive babies, we sometimes hear parents say, "My newborn FIGHTS sleep." Although this won't be true for the majority of babies, some do seem to fight sleep. They may cry even though you are holding them skin to skin, with a breast/bottle in their mouth, and rocking or using all of the Karp techniques! Some babies occasionally do seem to "blow off steam" by crying vigorously for 5-10 minutes before sleep. Some people would have you believe this is normal behavior for all babies. We believe it is normal behavior for some babies who are born with an intense temperament. We always encourage parents to soothe their babies, attempt to pinpoint a reason for the crying, and to refrain from assuming that their baby "needs" to cry. Most babies don't need to cry before sleep, but when an intense baby becomes over-stimulated or overly tired, he may fall asleep more quickly when most sources of stimulation are removed including rocking, feeding, and a parent's soothing noises.

Miriam shares:

Out of my five children, I've had two intense, easily overwhelmed babies. Neither of them had colic, but both could become overwhelmed easily. As a first time mom, I often remember thinking that Beka slept too much, and I couldn't wait for her to wake up to play! Beka and I would be having a wonderful time, smiling and laughing together. Her laughs would quickly turn to fussing one second and smiling the next. It was odd to watch, as she seemed to really enjoy interacting with me, but at the same time, she was feeling a bit overwhelmed. If I didn't go into sleepy mode right away the fussing would turn to screaming. Nothing would stop the crying. In fact, the more soothing I did, rocking, singing, offering a feeding, the more she cried. When I laid her down or put her in her swing, she would continue to cry, but then fall asleep within 5-10 minutes. Those few minutes felt like the longest of my life. It was SO hard to hear her cry, but at that point, she needed to shut out the world. She would then wake up refreshed and ready to play again. Thankfully, crying to sleep wasn't an everyday event. Most of the time, she went peacefully to sleep, in my arms or in her bassinet.

My fifth baby, Shannon, was also intense and perceptive, but by the time he came along, I had become more experienced in "Baby Talk." I noticed that he disliked some of my shirts. They were too busy and overwhelming for him, and if I wanted him to go to sleep or relax, I had to put on something with solid colors. With Shannon I used lots of skin to skin contact and baby wearing to keep him calm. I never needed to put him down to blow off steam.

More Techniques to Soothe Your Baby

Baby wearing: Some parents find that the only way to soothe a colicky baby is to hold and rock the baby constantly. Unfortunately, very few of us have time (or stamina) to actually do that! Baby wearing offers a nice compromise. With baby tucked safely in a sling, mom or dad can go about daily activities while still comforting baby. Baby wearing has been practiced all over the world, for probably most of human existence. It's a great way to protect, nurture, and interact with your baby. Be aware that there are many different types of wraps, baby carriers, and slings. Infant slings are not recommended for babies under 4 months of age, since they may not be able to keep their airways open in a sling. A wrap or infant carrier can be used instead. Talk to your health care provider, if you have any questions. You may want to try several different types of wraps and carriers before purchasing one; finding just the right carrier can make baby wearing much more enjoyable for you and your baby.

To make baby wearing as safe as possible, keep a few things in mind. When your baby is in the wrap or carrier make sure your baby's back is supported and not in a curved position that could make breathing difficult; the chin should be off of the chest, the sling tight against your body, and baby in sight at all times. Be aware of your baby's breathing and airway, taking care to keep it clear. Wrap your baby in such a way that you are able to kiss the top of his head, as it rests close to your chin.

Nicole shares:

With my first, I didn't use a carrier until he was big enough for a Baby Bjorn. However, with my second (and a toddler to chase around), I found a carrier to be great with my second son! My toddler would chase me around the kitchen while my younger son fell asleep (in about 3 minutes flat!) in the carrier.

Daily routine: Intense babies can benefit greatly from a regular, daily schedule and routine. While it's not appropriate to impose a by-the-clock schedule on a newborn, you can build predictable routines into your baby's daily activities. You'll find more on newborn schedules in the next section of the book.

Skin to skin contact: <u>The best way to soothe and stabilize an upset newborn is **skin to skin** contact.</u> Doctors and medical researchers support what moms around the world have known for centuries: when newborns are held skin-to-skin against their mothers, they tend to stop crying and calm down quickly.

Responding to Your Babies Needs: This one may seem obvious, but in some ways it's a little counter-intuitive. You may hear some people teach that if you respond quickly to your newborn, you are teaching him to be self-centered or that you are rewarding his crying. They stress doing everything on a schedule, so parents remain in control and decide when a need is met, but newborns can't relate to a parent's clock or understand their need for control, and they can only remember things for a few seconds. Newborns learn to deal with distress by self-soothing only AFTER they have learned that distress can be resolved. It takes newborns awhile to learn that hunger and other discomforts can be fixed by caregivers. When you help your baby resolve his discomfort when he cues for help, he learns resilience – distress can be overcome. First, he'll learn that discomfort doesn't last forever, then that you can help him when he sends you a cue, and finally, he'll develop the confidence to self-soothe. Parents who respond quickly to newborn cues end up with babies who cry less and are less demanding overall.

Miriam shares:

After having five children I can attest to the fact that your sweet, little newborn will quickly turn into an independent and possibly fearless toddler and child. So, enjoy this special time when you're the only one who can meet your baby's needs. There is so much giving to be done as a parent, but there's nothing in the world quite like it.

Nicole shares:

While some people believe you can spoil a newborn, it will take time for your baby's needs to turn to wants. You must satisfy all your baby's needs, so he or she can learn to trust you and learn your home/world is a safe place. It is only after your baby or toddler learns that he has opinions and wants do you have to worry about giving him 'too much' and, thus, spoiling him. Regardless, there is never 'too much' hugging and other affection to be given.

Baby Talk

Crying isn't the only sound your newborn makes. You may have noticed your newborn grunting or sighing while she sleeps; this is perfectly normal. Therefore, try not to rush to your baby's side at every little sound she makes, unless it's close to feeding time. If you do, you might accidentally wake up your sleeping baby, and that's not something any mom or dad wants to do! She may simply be transitioning through a sleep cycle. Instead, wait a few moments and she may settle back to a deeper sleep.

Your Newborn's Posture, Body Language and Reflexes

Did you know that you can tell a lot about how your newborn is feeling just by observing his body language? It's true! Your newborn's body language speaks volumes about his needs.

Your Newborn's Natural Posture

Your newborn baby's natural posture looks very different from yours. Newborns spend a lot of time curled up in the womb, so it's natural that they spend the first few months of life curled into a snug fetal position.

A newborn will naturally keep her elbows bent, and her hands up by her face. Her legs will be bent, with knees drawn up to her chest and feet crossed.

Your Newborn's Body Language

Watch your newborn's body language to help you determine how he's feeling, and what he needs.

If your newborn kicks her legs, it could mean that she's happy and enthusiastic. Sometimes, babies will kick when they see something interesting, or become excited. Watch her face to be sure; if she is smiling or wide-eyed, it's a good sign that she's feeling good. However, if your newborn is grimacing and fussing as she kicks, these could be early warning signs that she's upset; act on them, and work to make her more comfortable.

If your newborn looks away and won't make eye contact, it could mean that he's feeling a bit overwhelmed and needs some space. You may notice this happening if you, or another adult, gets close to his face.

If your newborn is staring off in space, it is likely that she's tired and ready for sleep. If she's also rubbing her eyes and starting to fuss, then act quickly and get her to sleep; when you ignore the early signs of sleepiness, she'll likely become upset, and it'll be harder to help her fall asleep later. Rubbing of the eyes and fussiness are signs that a baby is already overly tired.

If your newborn arches her back, it likely means she's upset (especially if she's crying or screaming as she does it)! Back arching is often the obvious cue that follows a series of smaller, more subtle cues, like eye rubbing. If your newborn is lying on his back, with arms outstretched and hands open and relaxed, it probably means he's relaxed.

If your newborn is pulling on/hitting her ears, it could mean that she's distressed and in pain. She may have gas or stomach discomfort, or she may have an ear infection. Watch her face closely; if she's grimacing or crying, take it as a sign that something's making her uncomfortable.

Your Newborn's Reflexes

A reflex refers to a behavior that's performed instinctively, without any conscious thought, in response to some kind of stimulation. Newborns have a few distinct reflexive behaviors, including rooting (to find the breast), sucking, and grasping (when something is placed in their outstretched palm).

In fact, newborn behavior in general is reflexive. This is why it's impossible to "spoil" a newborn -- newborns cry when they have a need, and not as a way to manipulate mom and dad into paying attention, or into picking them up. What's more, newborns don't develop habits, the way older babies and toddlers do. That's why you really don't need to worry too much about rocking or feeding your baby to sleep during the newborn phase; it isn't until he's a bit older (4 months and beyond) that this can become a habit for him. Although we don't worry about parent-dependent sleep props at this age, some babies don't need as many as others, and can transition smoothly without needing to change routines. Give your baby the soothing he needs as he transitions to sleep, but you may be surprised at how well he can fall asleep on his own, given the chance.

Remember, your newborn is far too young to cry in an effort to "make" you do something. Newborn babies don't have a sense of self like toddlers and adults do. They don't know that parents exist when they are out of sight. Newborns can only think of one thing at a time. For instance, you may see your baby hurt himself by scratching his face. He can only think of moving his hands; he can't organize his movements well or understand that his movements are causing the pain to his face. Here's another example, babies learn to pick up a rattle long before they learn to intentionally release it. This is because the grasping is reflexive and releasing is not reflexive. When you consider the reflexive nature of newborn behavior, it becomes clear that newborns can't intentionally manipulate their parents (although, it CAN feel that way!).

Here's a metaphor that may help you better understand your newborn's reflexive behavior. As an adult, you have reflexes, just like your newborn. For example, you have a blinking reflex that helps keep dust, dirt, and foreign objects out of your eyes. Your newborn's reflexive behaviors are just like your blinking reflex; they are automatic and beyond your baby's control. Expecting your newborn to stop her reflexive behaviors (crying, rooting, sucking her fingers, etc.) would be the same as expecting an adult to stop blinking in the middle of a dust storm.

After the newborn stage, later in infancy and into the toddler years, reflexive behaviors diminish as the brain has matured and developed the ability to perform intentional activities. Habits may have formed, and at this point, you may need to wean your baby away from sleep props (like rocking to sleep, swaddling, nursing to sleep, using the pacifier at night, etc.) In the newborn stage, these sleep props help babies transition between sleep and wake states; later, they become hindrances to sleep as babies wake between sleep cycles to ensure their props are in place.

How will you know it's time to wean from parent-dependent sleep props? Your baby will let you know. Instead of being rocked to sleep and then sleeping peacefully in his crib or beside you in bed, he'll wake up the second you lay him down or a few minutes later. He may begin to wake every 1-2 hours and then suck at the breast or on his pacifier for a minute or two and fall back to sleep. Parent-dependent sleep props make sense when they lead to restful sleep for babies and parents, and they stop making sense when the baby wakes during or between sleep cycles 5-10 times per night to recreate the exact environment in which he went to sleep. The time to wean from parent-dependent sleep props will vary from baby to baby. Some babies do fine all through infancy with parent-dependent sleep props, while others begin to have problems at 3-4 months. Part of our job at the Baby Sleep Site® is to help you navigate weaning from sleep props when your baby shows signs of needing a new routine.

Learning "Baby Talk" is a lot like learning a whole new language and culture. As you get to know your baby better each day, you'll begin to understand his vocalizations, reflexive cues, body posture, and cries. You'll begin to connect all of his baby "talk" to the contextual clues related to his activity cycles, and before you know it, you'll be an excellent communicator with your baby.

ESSENTIAL KEY #3: SCHEDULES AND SLEEP

A flexible schedule that allows your newborn's needs to be met while providing structure to sleep and wake patterns will help lay the foundation for healthy sleep habits later in life. If you tend to be a "Type A" person (one who's highly organized, and who likes to be in control), the word "schedule" is likely a happy one for you. However, if you tend to be more of a free spirit (a person who likes to go with the flow) then "schedule" might be a word that makes you crazy!

The good news is that there's no "correct" method of parenting out there. The way one family implements a schedule will look different than the way another family does it - and that's okay! The purpose of this section isn't to convince you to create a rigid schedule that your whole family must follow. At The Baby Sleep Site®, we understand that what works for one family won't necessarily work for another, and we're committed to respecting individual and family differences.

Rather, in this section of the book, we want to offer some information about the kind of sleep schedule and rhythms your newborn will fall into naturally, as well as some information about how you can create a flexible schedule that will work for your newborn and for you. Simply knowing what is normal and recognizing a newborn's natural rhythms can help parents feel more confident. Parents can also learn to respond proactively to a day's events by gently guiding their newborn through family activities.

To understand how a newborn's day works, we'll use the words schedule, activity cycle, and routine. The "schedule" refers to the "big picture" – the events of the entire 24 hour period like your normal morning wake-up time and bed time. The term "activity cycle" refers to the sleep and wake cycles that newborns experience many times per day. "Routine" indicates the way parents manage activity cycles and also the small steps cueing each new activity or transition between activities (for example, singing a lullaby before bedtime or feeding right before bedtime.)

Newborn Sleep/Wake Cycles

Newborns have activity cycles as they move through their day. Your baby's sleep/wake cycles will be fairly short in the days and weeks right after birth, but as he gets older, those activity cycles will begin to lengthen.

Typical Sleep/Wake Cycles for Newborns

In the first month or two after birth, your baby's sleeping schedule is driven by his feeding needs: he'll wake when he's hungry and fall asleep again when he's had enough to eat (and perhaps played a bit). So, a typical newborn sleep/wake cycle might look something like this:

- **Baby wakes up.** Newborns will wake anywhere from one to four hours after the start of their last feeding.

- **Baby eats.** Feedings can last anywhere from 20 minutes to an hour in the newborn stage. This depends on the type of feeding (bottle or breast) as well as on your baby's age (newborns tend to eat more slowly, but they'll learn to eat more quickly and efficiently as they grow).

- **Baby gets diaper change and/or bath.***

- **Baby "plays".*** Your newborn won't be up for any actual playing, but you can keep him awake for a bit after a feeding by engaging him in some tummy time, or by showing him some toys or reading a few books while he lies in your arms. This playtime will be fairly short in the early weeks after birth, but it will slowly get longer as your baby grows.

- **Baby goes back to sleep.** After feeding and playing, your newborn will be ready to go back to sleep. This sleep may be fairly short (as short as half an hour) or relatively long (as long as 2 hours).

*Activities and playtime should be included in your baby's daytime activity cycle, but not in her nighttime cycles. At night, feed your baby and then put her right back to bed.

While this is considered a typical example of a newborn's sleep/wake cycle, don't be concerned if your newborn doesn't follow this pattern perfectly. You may find that your newborn sleeps for long stretches at some points of the day, and then takes a series of mini-naps at other points in the day. Some feedings may take longer, while other times, your newborn may take in several, "snack-y" feedings in a short time.

This is all very normal. Remember, your newborn will need to eat more frequently during a growth spurt (see page 70), and that may mean her sleep is more broken up than usual during these phases. Or, as your newborn grows, he may start to sleep longer stretches at night and then take shorter naps (and feed more often) during the day. Again - normal.

As your baby grows, and as he starts to distinguish days from nights, these sleep cycles will change. Your baby will start to spend more time awake during the day, and more time asleep at night.

Miriam shares:

My mother was amazing with Beka. She helped so much the first few days after Beka's birth and while I was recovering. I wondered if I would ever be able to understand my baby's cues as well as she did. Mom had four children, and had lots of practice in 'Baby Talk.' A few months later, she was watching Beka for a few hours, and I came back to find Beka crying. I knew exactly what she needed. My mom asked, 'How did you know?' After working with many first time moms and babies, I now know the answer to that question - it's because I was Beka's mommy, and our relationship born of love and time spent together couldn't be replaced by anyone else. The same is true for you and your baby, even if it doesn't feel like it at first. There will never be anyone who understands your baby as well as you do!

Day/Night Confusion

One of the most frustrating elements of parenting a newborn is the day/night confusion that many newborn babies experience. If only our babies came out of the womb understanding that nighttime is for sleeping! Unfortunately, they don't.

Your newborn's nighttime waking will largely be due to his need to eat every few hours, but many newborns experience excessive nighttime waking. Parents of these newborns report that their newborns' longer, 3-4 hour periods of sleep are happening during the day, while their periods of frequent eating and catnapping are happening at night. If your newborn fits this description, it may feel like your baby has his days and nights completely reversed!

Why Do Newborns Mix Up Their Days and Nights?

Not to worry; day/night confusion is normal for newborns. During pregnancy, a baby's sleeping rhythms are closely tied to mom's rhythms. This is due, at least in part, to the fact that a pregnant mom's hormones are passed to her baby, so when mom's body is releasing melatonin (the hormone that helps us sleep), baby's rhythms are affected. After birth, however, this link between mom and baby is broken, unless mom is breastfeeding. Furthermore, when you were pregnant, your movement during the day likely lulled your baby to sleep (imagine lying on a boat docked in the ocean all day and being lulled to sleep by the waves). I'm sure you remember your baby may have woken up to party just as you were lying down to go to sleep at night (and the movement stopped). This led to her being more awake at night and sleeping for much of the day.

Circadian rhythms refer to the roughly 24-hour internal clock that we adults all have. This internal clock is heavily influenced by sunlight; when we're exposed to sunlight, it helps our clocks to know that it's time to wake up, and when it's dark outside, it tells our clocks that it's time to go to sleep.

Once your baby is born, he begins to rely on his own internal clock to tell him when it's time to be awake and when it's time to sleep. Every cell in our bodies has a clock, and it takes time for a newborn to synchronize his clocks with the outside world. This is another reason why he may be wide awake in the middle of the night, and sleeping soundly in the middle of the afternoon.

Resolving Your Newborn's Day/Night Confusion

There's no quick fix for day/night confusion. While this can feel frustrating to exhausted parents of newborns, rest assured that even if you don't do a thing to correct it, most of the time this problem will eventually sort itself out. Day/Night confusion is often resolved by 8 weeks. At about 3 months of age, your baby's melatonin production will start to become more like yours, and by 5 or 6 months of age, her circadian rhythms will be more fully developed. All of this will help her sleep longer at night and less during the day.

While there's no fast way to resolve the problem, there are a few things you can do to help gently encourage your newborn to sleep more during nighttime hours and less during daylight hours:

- **Wake your baby occasionally during the day, if he's sleeping for long periods of time.** You may have heard the old saying, "Never wake a sleeping baby." While we generally agree with this adage, there are exceptions, and this is one of them. In order to help your newborn sort out day and night, he needs to be awake during the day for his circadian rhythms to adjust to life outside the womb. Therefore, it's best to limit any one nap to two hours, and to keep your baby awake after each daytime feeding, even if it's only for a few minutes. This will help "reset" his clock.

- **Expose your baby to sunlight during the day.** We're not talking about direct, outside sunlight here; do that, and your baby could suffer from sunburn! However, it is important to make sure that your baby doesn't spend all her time in a dim room, with the shades drawn. Instead, during the day, try feeding her and playing with her in a sunny room in the house; until day/night confusion is resolved, daytime naps should take place in a sunny room as well. Then, when it's time to sleep at night, put her in a very dark room (try some room-darkening shades or blackout liners). Being exposed to sunlight and darkness like this will help guide her circadian rhythms in the right direction.

- **Make days "exciting" and nights "boring".** When your baby wakes from a nap during the day, encourage his awake time by doing something stimulating, like playing with a toy, reading a book, giving a bath, etc. This will help promote daytime wakefulness. In contrast, keep nighttime stimulation to a minimum. When your baby wakes at night, feed him quietly. Keep his room dark, turning on only as much light as you need to feed and tend to him. Make his diaper change brief. Then, put him right back to sleep.

Resolving Day/Night Confusion: What Not to Do!

It should be noted that there are also a few "don'ts" when it comes to solving your newborn's day/night confusion:

- **NEVER withhold a feeding from your newborn, in an attempt to make her sleep longer at night.** Remember, your newborn needs to eat frequently. A newborn shouldn't go more than 2-3 hours without a feeding, with maybe one four hour stretch at night during a 24 hour period.

- **NEVER let your newborn cry it out.** A newborn isn't always capable of self-soothing which is necessary for doing any real sleep training; that needs to wait until he's older.

- **Don't keep your baby awake for long periods of time during the day, in an attempt to make him sleep longer at night.** While it's fine to occasionally wake your baby from a long daytime nap, don't keep your newborn awake for hours on end, in the hopes that doing so will make him sleep better at night. Do this, and your newborn will become overtired. And contrary to what you might expect, an overtired baby will actually sleep less than a baby who's well-rested!

Managing Twins and Multiples

Having one newborn can be overwhelming in and of itself -- but having 2 or 3 or more!? That's a giant task indeed! While the newborn stage will definitely be more challenging when you have twins or multiples, there are some steps you can take, right from the beginning, to help things go more smoothly.

Utilizing Tandem Schedules

When you have newborn twins or multiples, it's helpful to keep tandem schedules -- make sure that all babies are doing the same thing at the same time. This means that if one baby wakes to feed, go ahead and feed the other. Do diaper changes, feedings, naps, etc. at the same time for each baby. This approach does not always work forever and there will be times when you will need to stagger your babies' schedules (see the next section for details). But in the beginning, it's important to do what you need to in order to get through each day, and keeping your babies on the same schedule will really help!

It's also important to note that, while most newborns aren't ready for by-the-clock schedules, when you have twins, you might want to stick to a more clock-based schedule for sanity sake. This will help greatly in keeping both babies on the same schedule.

Utilizing Staggered Schedules

There may be times when, instead of keeping your babies on a tandem schedule, you need to stagger your babies' schedules, and do each babies' daily activities at different times. Staggering your babies' schedules by even 15 minutes can work. Times to use staggered schedules include...

- ...when one baby is ill. If one baby becomes ill, then the other baby may get sick, too. But if just one baby is ill, you may need to adjust that baby's schedule, to allow for more sleep and more feedings.

- ...when one baby clearly has a higher sleep need than the other. Again, in the early weeks after delivery, it's probably best to use a tandem schedule as much as possible (to maintain your own sanity)! But as your babies get a bit older, if it becomes clear that one has different sleep needs than the other, you can modify the sleep schedules a bit, to compensate.

- ...if you want to spend time with your babies one-on-one. If you feel like you aren't spending enough time with your babies individually, try staggering their schedules for a day or two, in order to get more one-on-one time.

- ...if you are ready to start sleep coaching. When you are ready to help your babies learn to fall asleep on their own, it can help to stagger their schedules. This way, you can work on sleep coaching with one baby at a time.

Separate Sleep Spaces

Sometimes multiples will be so different that it can work much better to have them sleep in separate rooms, if possible. We work with many parents with multiples, and many times one sleeps much better than the other, but when they are sleeping in the same room, both or all are disturbed when one wakes. The easiest solution when families have limited space, and have chosen to have their babies sleep in their nursery is for one baby to sleep in a pack-n-play in the living area or parent's room or other space (one mom we worked with used a walk-in closet!) while another sleeps in the nursery until both or all are sleeping better at night.

Asking for Help with Twins and Multiples

Having outside help is important for all parents of newborns, but it's downright crucial for parents of multiples! So don't hesitate to ask friends and family members to come over and help you with the babies. The extra hands will go a long way towards helping you enjoy the early weeks after delivery. See additional tips for asking for help on Page 61.

Your Baby's Changing Sleep Patterns

For the first few weeks of your baby's life, your baby will probably wake for feedings fairly consistently, around the clock. At this stage, babies need to eat about every 3-4 hours during the night (although a small percentage of newborns 6-8 weeks old may be able to stretch that closer to 5 or 6 hours at night.) While it's true that some 8 week old babies can sleep 7 or 8 hours at night, without needing to eat, this is far from standard. The majority of 8 week old babies need to eat at least once (probably 2 or 3 times) during a 10 hour night.

Between 8 and 12 weeks of age, many babies gradually start sleeping a bit longer at night. You may notice that your baby consistently has a long period of sleep at night (5 or 6 hours, for example). You may also notice that your baby is awake a bit more during the day. These are a good signs; it means that your baby's internal clock and hormone production is developing. This is also the point at which your baby may be technically "sleeping through the night" (since sleeping through the night is defined as 5 straight hours of sleep, with no feedings).

Between 12 and 16 weeks of age, your baby's sleep patterns will change permanently. Whereas your baby probably fell asleep quickly and slept very deeply in the newborn stage, by 3 or 4 months of age, your baby will start to cycle in and out of deep and light sleep, just like we adults do.

What does this mean? It means that while your 3 or 4 month old is capable of sleeping longer stretches at night, and feeding less often, <u>she may still wake often at night, even though she's not actually hungry at each waking.</u> This night waking will happen during her lighter periods of sleep, when she's coming out of one sleep cycle and ready to start another. Your baby may wake during these transitions, and if she's used to having you around to put her to sleep, she'll cry for you to come and help her fall back to sleep. During this stage (around 4 months), you can start trying some gentle sleep coaching with your baby.

Foundation for Healthy Sleep Habits

Your baby isn't ready for a strict, by-the-clock schedule. However, this doesn't mean that you can't encourage your newborn to follow a gentle, flexible schedule.

Many babies will gradually develop their own schedule in the first 12 weeks of life. (Not every baby will do this, however, so don't stress if your baby doesn't!) If you notice some predictable patterns emerging in your baby's behavior, encourage those patterns. Try watching for his hunger and sleep cues; when you see them, act quickly. This will help you stay ahead of any overtiredness, and will ensure that your baby is well-rested.

Some babies will need a bit more coaxing and direction from mom and dad in order to develop a schedule. While your baby isn't ready for any strict sleep schedule, there are a few gentle methods and techniques you can use to help encourage a healthy sleep schedule for your newborn. These methods are gentle enough to be used at any time during the newborn period, as long as you keep in mind that neither the caregiver nor the baby should feel distressed when using them.

Gentle Methods to Shift Sleep

The Fading Method

This is a no-cry (or very little cry) gentle sleep coaching method. With the fading method, you help your baby fall asleep, but you set up "rules" as to how you will slowly take yourself out of the equation. If you think about how you have done most of the work up until this point, now you will develop rules to follow that will shift the "work" to your baby.

For example, if you have always rocked baby all the way to sleep, you might rock her a bit less and put her in the crib drowsy but awake, and let her try to fall asleep on her own. If she gets worked up, you try to quiet and soothe her using other methods (like patting, a tummy rub, or shushing) until she is asleep. As time passes, you should slowly do less and less "work" and your baby should do more of it.

This is a great method to use when your baby is young, since it involves little to no crying and still leaves plenty of room for you to meet baby's needs. We don't expect fast results, but after a week or so of effort at bedtime and/or after working on at least, two naps per day, you should see consistent improvement.

Nicole shares:

This method has the possibility of being very gentle, depending on your baby's temperament and how accepting she is of alternative soothing methods. It can, however, take the patience of Job. My son took two long hours the first night. I was able to limit his fussing and crying by laying him next to me and soothing him in other ways, but letting him do the "work" of falling asleep, in the end. It took a lot of patience, because I knew if I just breastfed or rocked him, he'd be asleep in two minutes! I thought it would be faster the second night, but no! It took two hours, again. However, on the third night, he did it in just 20 minutes and this foundation led the way to much better sleep for all of us! My persistence and commitment really paid off. If this method does not lead to limited crying, take a break and then try again. Even failed attempts does not mean your baby is not learning. Just think of how many times he will fall before he successfully walks!

The "Pick-Up-Put-Down" Method (PUPD)

This method is discussed by Tracy Hogg in her book, *Secrets of The Baby Whisperer*. The PUPD method works just the way it sounds: when it's time to sleep, and your baby is fussing in his crib or bassinet, you pick him up and comfort him until he's calm and drowsy. Then, you put him back in his crib to sleep, repeating this cycle until your baby is finally asleep. With a newborn this may take 30 minutes of consistent work (about 3-4 pick up and put down cycles). It is usually best to pick 1-2 times per day to try this, because using it at all sleep times is too stressful for baby. Some families will find the most success working only on bedtime for 3-4 days and then moving on to two of the 5-6 naps, once bedtime is going smoothly.

It's important to note that the PUPD method won't work for every baby (or every parent, for that matter). Some babies find being picked up and put down often way too stimulating; for those babies, the PUPD method ends up being upsetting instead of soothing. If you decide to try this approach with your baby, stop quickly if you find your baby becoming increasingly upset or increase the amount of time you spend soothing your baby while holding her. To use this method, you may need to begin by putting your baby down when very, very drowsy, and work your way toward putting her down from a more awake state over a period of time. The eventual goal is to put her down when she is drowsy, but awake enough to realize she is settling to sleep independently.

Miriam shares:

I used the pick up/put down method with my third baby, Eli. It took maybe 15 minutes the first time I tried it. I used it as soon as we got home from the hospital for a couple of his daily naps. I would put him down just the tiniest bit awake; he would make little noises, wiggle around, and then scrunch up his face to cry. I would pick him up, feed him for a few seconds, rock him, and put him back down, again just the tiniest bit awake. After 3 or 4 tries it worked! For his other naps, I would hold him, rock him, feed him, put him in a baby carrier, or occasionally swaddle him, and put him in his swing with a pacifier. I had a preschooler and a toddler at the time, so it was nice that he could take a few of his naps independently. Eli was a big baby and due to my milk supply and his size, he needed to be fed every 2 hours around the clock for the first 6 weeks. Because, I was spending so much time feeding, those few naps in his bed and swing helped me manage the rest of my day.

Establishing Fixed Points

A Fixed Point is a tool to help you add some predictability to your days. Fixed Points can be very helpful to your baby as well! We encourage moms to consider having a few Fixed Points in their "normal" day. We know that it can feel like no two days are alike and that "normal" days can seem all too elusive, but maybe they'll become a little more of a regular occurrence, if you use a few Fixed Points. Keep in mind that Fixed Points are a tool for you! Don't feel like you HAVE to use them, or that you've failed if you don't meet them; they are simply a tool to help you order your day, if that is important to you.

Fixed Point One: Establishing a Consistent Morning Wake-Up Time

A great way to help your newborn work towards a consistent schedule is to wake your newborn at roughly the same time each morning (within 30 minutes or so). If your baby wakes at a consistent time each morning, it'll be easier to keep her daytime feedings and sleep consistent and fairly predictable. If your baby wakes at different times each morning, however, it can be hard to develop a schedule.

It's best if you track your baby's morning wake time for a week or so, to see if there's a pattern. If you notice that your baby generally wakes at a specific time, encourage that pattern by making sure that you wake your baby within 30 minutes of that time each morning. However, use your judgment when using this technique; if your baby has a rough night, it may be best to let him sleep a bit longer.

Fixed Point Two: Establishing an Appropriate Bedtime

Having a consistent morning wake-up time is key to establishing a predictable schedule for your baby; so is having a consistent bedtime. However, should you make your newborn's bedtime later in the evening, in an attempt to help her "sleep in?" Or is an earlier bedtime better?

In the first 6 weeks of your baby's life, you'll probably find that the concept of bedtime doesn't really apply to your baby's days and nights. After all, at this stage, your baby is eating every few hours, around the clock, so there's nothing really distinct about daytime vs. nighttime. During this stage, you may try to time up your baby's bedtime with your own -

maybe by feeding baby right before you're ready to go to sleep yourself. This works well in the newborn stage, and helps you maximize your own nighttime sleep. In fact, some moms find it helpful to become a bit of a night owl. Some newborns are prone to nursing the most between 9 pm and 12 am. If you tend to enjoy sleeping in, the newborn stage is the time to indulge!

However, after the newborn stage is over, you'll want to start working towards establishing a separate bedtime for your baby. By 3 or 4 months, your baby will likely be feeding 2-3 times per night (or perhaps just once), and enjoying an 11-12 hour night, while feeding more often and sleeping less during the day. This means you'll be able to better distinguish and separate your baby's days and nights.

What's more, once you've reached the 3-4 month mark and are ready to work towards a separate bedtime for baby, you'll want to make sure that bedtime is fairly early. It might seem like a later bedtime would be a better idea; after all, won't a baby who's gone to sleep later in the evening wake up later in the morning?

The answer is almost always no; baby sleep doesn't work that way. In reality, an early bedtime is crucial to a good night's sleep once you leave the newborn stage. When babies and young children are overtired, they may have more difficulty falling asleep and staying asleep and will often wake too early in the morning. While many parents think that keeping a child up later at night is best, it's actually the early bedtime that will lead to a more restful sleep and a later waking in the morning once you leave the newborn stage. You'll know it's time to transition to an earlier bedtime when your baby's last catnap extends to an hour or more. That's the first clue that he is ready for a longer night. You may be able to move that catnap 15-30 minutes later in the evening and it will merge with bedtime. At 3-4 months we expect bedtime to occur between 6:30 and 8:00 pm.

Developing a schedule for a newborn is as easy as identifying a consistent bedtime (whether that is 11:00 pm in the early days or 7:00 pm by 16 weeks), a consistent morning wake-up time, and a consistent first nap and first afternoon nap. All other nap times and night waking times may vary according to your baby's changing needs, but having 3 or 4 points of certainty in your day can make a big difference for parent and baby! These "fixed points" aren't necessarily rigid, by the clock times, but having them in mind and trying to follow them on most days can be very helpful to some parents and babies.

We wanted to provide you with some hypothetical days, so you will have an idea of what your day may look like with a newborn. You'll see the word "wake" on the schedule. This indicates the time the baby woke from sleep, not a time the parent woke him. Also, the "Description" indicates how long you can expect the baby to be awake in each time slot, but keep in mind, newborns will sometimes surprise you with a short cat nap long before they are "due" for their next nap or they may sleep longer than you expect and that's okay as well. At this age we want to establish a few fixed points, but every day will likely be slightly different the first few months.

Sample Daily Routines

Weeks 2-8: This might be what a day would look like for a breastfeeding mom with a small storage capacity and/or a baby with reflux.

Time	Description	Notes
9:00 am	Wake and Feed *(fixed point)	Try to begin every day within 30 minutes of 'wake-up time.'
10:00 am	Nap (45 min -1 hour awake) *fixed point	~30-60 minutes
11:00 am	Wake and feed	
12:00 pm	Nap (1 - 1 ½ hours awake)	~30-60 minutes
12:30 pm	Wake and feed	
1:30 pm	Feed (snack) and Nap	~20-30 minutes
1:50 pm	Wake	If still sleeping, do not wake!
2:30 pm	Feed *	
3:15 pm	Nap (1 ½ to 2 hours awake) *	~30 - 60 minutes
4:00 pm	Wake and Feed	
5:00 pm	Nap (1 ½ to 2 hours awake)	~30-60 minutes
6:00 pm	Wake and Feed	
7:30 pm	Feed	
8:00 pm	Nap (1 ½ to 2 hours awake)	~30-60 minutes

8:30 pm	Wake and feed	
9:30 pm	Feed *	
10:00 pm	Bedtime *	
12:00 am	Feed and back to sleep	
4:00 am	Feed and back to sleep	
7:00 am	Feed and back to sleep	

Looking at the hypothetical day above, you may wonder why we labeled some feeding times as fixed points. Newborns will usually take a feeding (maybe only a small feeding) whenever one is offered, especially if mom uses breast compressions to increase milk flow, and we know that feedings and sleep are connected. The chances of getting sleep at fixed points during a day are better when a feeding is offered beforehand. You'll notice there was no feeding offered prior to the morning nap. Although some babies will need a feeding before this nap, many will be able to go to sleep without one, since the first feeding of the day is usually a "larger" feeding.

2-8 weeks: Breastfeeding Mom with average storage capacity and average milk supply, baby without reflux.

Time	Description	Notes
9:00 am	Wake and Feed	
10:00 am	Nap	~30-60 minutes
11:00 am	Wake and Feed	
12:30 pm	Nap (1 ½ hours awake)	~30-60 minutes
1:30 pm	Wake and Feed	
3:30 pm	Nap (1 ½ to 2 hours awake)	~30 - 60 minutes
4:30 pm	Wake and Feed	
6:00 pm	Nap (1 ½ to 2 hours awake)	~30 - 60 minutes
6:30 pm	Wake and Feed	
7:30 pm	Catnap (1 ½ to 2 hours awake)	~30 – 60 minutes
8:00 pm	Wake and Feed	
9:30 pm	Catnap (1 to 2 hours awake)	~ 20-30 minutes
10:00 pm	Wake and Feed	
11:30 pm	Feed and Bedtime	
3:30 am	Feed and sleep	
6:30 am	Feed and sleep	

2-8 Weeks: Breastfeeding Mom with a large storage capacity and baby with a large stomach capacity.

Time	Description	Notes
9:00 am	Wake and Feed	
10:00 am	Nap (1 hour awake)	~60-90 minutes
11:30 am	Wake	
12:30 pm	Feed and Nap (1 hour awake)	~30 - 60 minutes
1:30 pm	Wake	
3:00 pm	Feed and Nap (1 to 1 ½ hours awake)	~60 - 90 minutes
4:30 pm	Wake and Feed	
6:00 pm	Nap (1 ½ to 2 hours awake)	~ 30-60 minutes
6:30 pm	Wake	
7:30 pm	Feed and Nap (1 to 2 hours awake)	~30-60 minutes
8:30 pm	Wake	
9:30 pm	Nap	~30-60 minutes
10:00 pm	Wake and Feed	
11:30 pm	Feed and Bedtime	
4:30 am	Feed and Sleep	
7:30 am	Feed and Sleep	

Possible day at 8-16 weeks: Breastfeeding Mom with smaller storage capacity and/or a baby who needs to eat more frequently.

Time	Description	Notes
7:00 am	Wake and Feed	
8:30 am	Nap (1 ½ hours awake)	~30-90 minutes
9:00 am	Wake and Feed	
11:00 am	Feed and Nap (1 ½ to 2 hours awake)	~30 - 120 minutes
1:00 pm	Wake and Feed	
2:00 pm	Nap (1 to 1 ½ hours awake)	~30 - 60 minutes
2:30 pm	Wake and Feed	
4:30 pm	Feed and Nap	~30-90 minutes
6:00 pm	Wake and Feed	
7:30 pm	Feed and Catnap (1 ½ to 2 hours awake)	~30 minutes
8:00 pm	Wake and Feed	
9:30 pm	Feed and Bedtime (1 ½ to 2 hours awake)	~30 minutes
11:00 pm	Dream Feed	(dream feeds should always take place at Mom's bedtime, so mom gets a long stretch of sleep; be sure to use breast compressions at bedtime and night feedings)
5:00 am	Wake and Feed	

8-16 Weeks: Breastfeeding Mom with average storage capacity and Baby with average stomach size.

Time	Description	Notes
7:00 am	Wake and Feed	
8:30 am	Nap (1 ½ hours awake)	~60-90 minutes
10:00 am	Wake and Feed	
11:30 am	Nap (1 ½ hours awake)	~60-90 minutes
1:00 pm	Wake and Feed	
2:30 pm	Nap (1 ½ to 2 hours awake)	~30 - 60 minutes
3:00 pm	Wake and Feed	
4:30 pm	Catnap (1 ½ to 2 hours awake)	30 minutes
5:00 pm	Wake and Feed	
6:30 pm	Catnap (1 ½ to 2 hours awake)	30 minutes
7:00 pm	Wake and Feed	
9:00 pm	Feed and Bedtime	
10:30 pm	Dream Feed	
2:00 am	Feed and Sleep	

8-16 Weeks: Breastfeeding Mom with larger storage capacity and baby who can take 4 or more ounces per feeding.

Time	Description	Notes
7:00 am	Wake and Feed	
8:30 am	Nap (1 ½ hours awake)	~60-90 minutes
10:00 am	Wake and Feed	
11:30 am	Nap (1 ½ to 2 hours awake)	~60 - 90 minutes
1:00 pm	Wake and Feed	
2:30 pm	Nap (1 ½ to 2 hours awake)	~60 minutes
3:30 pm	Wake	
4:00 pm	Nurse	
4:30 pm	Catnap (1 to 2 hours awake)	~30 minutes
5:00 pm	Wake	
6:00 pm	Feed	
6:30 pm	Nap	~20-30 minutes
8:30 pm	Feed and Bedtime	
10:00 pm	Dream Feed	
5:00 am	Feed and Sleep	

2-8 Weeks with a formula fed baby:

Time	Description	Notes
9:00 am	Wake and Feed* **(fixed point)**	
10:00 am	Nap (1 hour awake)	~60-90 minutes
11:30 am	Wake	
12:30 pm	Feed* and Nap (1 hour awake)	~30 - 60 minutes
1:30 pm	Wake	
3:00 pm	Feed and Nap (1 to 1 ½ hours awake)	~60 - 90 minutes
4:30 pm	Wake and Feed*	
6:00 pm	Nap (1 ½ to 2 hours awake)	~ 30-60 minutes
6:30 pm	Wake	
7:30 pm	Feed and Nap (1 to 2 hours awake)	~30-60 minutes
8:30 pm	Wake	
9:30 pm	Nap	~30-60 minutes
10:00 pm	Wake and Feed	
11:30 pm	Feed* and Bedtime	
4:30 am	Feed and Sleep	
7:30 am	Feed and Sleep	

9-14 Weeks for a formula feeding baby:

Time	Description	Notes
7:00 am	Wake and Feed	
8:30 am	Nap (1 ½ hours awake)	~60-90 minutes
10:00 am	Wake and Feed	
11:30 am	Nap (1 ½ to 2 hours awake)	~60 - 90 minutes
1:00 pm	Wake and Feed	
2:30 pm	Nap (1 ½ to 2 hours awake)	~60 minutes
3:30 pm	Wake	
4:00 pm	Feed	
4:30 pm	Catnap (1 to 2 hours awake)	~30 minutes
5:00 pm	Wake	
6:00 pm	Feed	
6:30 pm	Nap	~20-30 minutes
8:30 pm	Feed and Bedtime	
10:00 pm	Dream Feed	
5:00 am	Feed and Sleep	

15-20 Weeks with formula feeding baby:

Time	Description	Notes
6:30am	Wake and Feed	
7:30/7:45am	Nap (1 to 1 ½ hours awake)	~60+ minutes (ideally)
9:00/9:30 am	Feed	
9:30/10:00am	Nap (1 ½ hours awake)	~30 - 60 minutes
11:30/12:30pm	Feed and Nap (1 ½ to 2 hours awake)	~30 - 45 minutes, usually
~3:00pm	Feed and catnap (1 ½ to 2 hours awake)	~30 minutes, usually
5:00pm	Begin cluster-feeding to see if he will take more formula	
5:30/6:00pm	Begin bedtime routine	Use the earlier time if he doesn't take a fourth nap, takes all short naps, or skips a nap
5:45/6:15pm	Last feed, bedtime and lights out	
6:00/6:30pm	Goal to be asleep	

As you can see, one baby's day may look very different than another's! Accepting the baby and the body we have and then adjusting days to make it all work is one of the big jobs of motherhood. It can be frustrating if you hear about friends who are getting 6-8 hours of sleep at night when you're still getting up every 2-4 hours. Thankfully, this time of frequent feedings and many night wakings lasts only a few months.

Prioritizing Your Sleep, and Asking for Help

Of course, in order to stay healthy (and sane!) you'll want to prioritize your own sleep schedule, too. One way to do this is to avoid any impulses to be an 'overachieving' new parent. Remember, during the newborn stage, feeding and caring for your baby is practically a full-time job! So give yourself a break, and let non-essential things go. Your sleep, and your baby's sleep, are far more important than the cleaning and cooking and laundry! You can deal with those things in a few months, when you're past the newborn stage.

You can also prioritize your sleep - and your sanity - by accepting (and asking for) help. Just be sure that the help you ask for and receive is truly helpful! A well-meaning grandmother may want to 'help' by holding and playing with the baby, but if she keeps the baby awake too long, that won't be helpful at all. But maybe, in this instance, you could ask grandma to come over and hold the baby during his evening fussy time, so that you can eat something.

And remember, your helpers don't always have to be helping with the baby. In fact, it may be better for everyone if your helpers focus on things like cleaning and cooking and errand-running; that will free you up to care for your baby. Close friends and family members who truly do want to help won't mind helping in these ways.

Nicole shares:

All of us will have a different definition of what a "great parent" is, but I think we can all agree that being tired doesn't always bring out the greatness. I had a mom e-mail me once that both her kids outgrew their sleep problems around two and she said that, to her, it is just a "season of sleep deprivation" that will go away, eventually. She implied there wasn't much of a reason to "work" on it, if it will end on its own, anyway (even if it's years later). My challenge to her is that yes, SOME will have kids that outgrow these issues, but tell that to the parents with a five year old in their bed. Yes, eventually, perhaps even that five year old will outgrow it. But, whether it's 3 months, 12 months, 2 years, 5 years or 8 years, how many missed opportunities will you have to be a great mom or dad? So, be sure to take advantage of the opportunities you have to bond with your baby and get some extra sleep for yourself by taking advantage of the help your friends and family offer that way you can cherish those special (and fleeting) moments with your newborn. Sometimes I have looked so forward to bedtime and I kick myself because I know they won't be this little forever. One day they will be too busy with their friends to bother with mom (sniff sniff). I want to cherish it. Don't you?

Managing Older Children When You Have a Newborn

Simply feeding and caring for a baby who is just a few weeks old can be quite time consuming But newborn care is made even more challenging when you have older children to care for, too - particularly if you have toddlers and preschoolers at home.

Toddlers and preschoolers may (understandably) feel left out during feeding time - mom or dad is totally focused on the new baby, and that can feel frustrating or unsettling to a toddler or preschooler (especially since the older child may already be struggling with feelings of displacement, now that there is a new baby in the family).

Don't be surprised if your toddler or preschooler tends to act up during feedings. Acting out is likely her way of ensuring that you pay attention her, too. You can be proactive by ensuring that she has plenty to do, to keep her occupied during feeding times.

In the early days, when you and your baby are still sorting out the mechanics of feeding you will likely need both hands at feeding time - meaning you won't have a free hand for your toddler. You can compensate for this by doing some pre-feed planning. First, get your toddler settled and playing with some interesting books and toys. (Tip: consider having a 'special' box of toys that your toddler is only allowed to open during feeding time. This is a great way to make feeding time something that your toddler actually looks forward to!) Once your toddler is playing, be sure to either close the door to the room or put a gate across the doorway before you settle in to feed. This way, you ensure that you can supervise your toddler carefully while feeding -- you don't want your toddler choosing that particular moment to take a tumble down the stairs, or to run outside!

Later, when feeding is easier for both you and your new baby, you will probably be able to do it one-handed. At that point, invite your toddler to sit with you at feeding time. Read a book or do a simple puzzle together, as you feed your newborn. This creates a nice way for you to spend quality time with your older child while simultaneously caring for your newborn.

You may be able to handle things differently with your preschooler (depending on your preschooler's disposition and temperament). Sometimes, preschoolers are eager to be helpers; if this is the case with your preschooler, encourage this desire by making him your 'feeding time helper'. Put him in charge of bringing you the burp cloth, for instance, or tell him that it's his job to sing the baby a song during feedings. Allow him to hold the bottle (if applicable and with your help!) and help you with burping.

Miriam shares:

It's pretty common for young children to express interest in breastfeeding again, especially if you nursed during part of your pregnancy. Some moms do nurse both an infant and a toddler, and this is fine as long as the infant has access to the colostrum in the first few days and then gets 'first dibs' at feeding times and is gaining weight appropriately. Sometimes a toddler will simple nestle against the breast to feel close to mom. One mom I know had an abundant milk supply and she would pump about 12 ounces each morning, and feed it to her 18 month old in a bottle or sippy cup and then breastfeed her infant throughout the day. It's pretty common for a 3 year old to try out breastfeeding and then decide they want the 'big kid milk' instead. Toddlers may simply want the opportunity to nurse once or twice a day for a few minutes. It's very common for them to do the things they see the baby getting a lot of attention doing. If they see the new baby getting a lot of attention while breastfeeding they may try breastfeeding, or if they see the baby getting a lot of attention while doing some other behavior they may try out those behaviors as well. It can be really helpful to give lots of affirmation for all of the big kid things the older sibling can do. Take time to really notice them for doing little things that the baby can't do. You could say, 'Wow! You can climb into your chair all by yourself, and the baby can't even sit in a chair yet; thank you for showing him how it's done. You have grown so big and strong!

Managing Different Nap Schedules

One of the toughest things about having multiple children to care for is juggling multiple nap schedules. Your newborn's nap needs are obviously very different than your toddler's. And it may feel, at first, like your newborn and your toddler are sleeping at completely different times -- making it impossible for you to take a quick nap (or do much of anything)!

Thankfully, with a little work on your part, you should be able to coordinate your toddler's afternoon nap with at least one of your newborn's naps. You can achieve this by making your toddler's nap time a fixed point in your newborn's afternoon schedule, and then timing the rest of your newborn's naps and feeds around that fixed point. See page 48 for information on "Fixed Points."

For instance, if your toddler typically naps from 1-3 p.m., then do your best to feed your newborn around 12:30 or so (more like 12:15 in those early days of feeding, when feedings typically take longer). Then, when your newborn is done eating, put both your toddler and your newborn down for a nap. Ideally, this will give you some time to yourself, to either catch up on your sleep (that's what we recommend!) or to catch up on other things.

If your toddler or preschooler doesn't nap anymore, though, it can be tough to carve out any time for yourself. You can compensate for this by instituting a 'rest time' at some point during the day. Rest time is essentially just quiet time that your toddler or preschooler spends in his room, playing with toys, looking at books, doing puzzles, or listening to music. Try to time up rest time with one of your newborn's naps, so that you get a short break during the day to relax a little.

Managing Your Older Child's Feelings

Suddenly having a new sibling at home is a pretty earth-shattering experience for your toddler or preschooler (particularly if your toddler or preschooler was an only child before). Here are just a few of the ways your older child may react to the new baby:

- She may be jealous of the new baby.

- She may be angry at the new baby, or at you and your partner – almost the way you would feel, if your partner brought home someone else. "What is wrong with me, wasn't I enough?"

- She may begin to misbehave and act out more than usual, and be more demanding (this is usually an attention-getting strategy).

- If she was looking forward to a sibling, she may be disappointed that the new baby can't play with her, or do the activities that she enjoys.

Remember, while these reactions can be frustrating to us as parents, they are perfectly understandable, when you consider things from your toddler or preschooler's perspective. The best thing you can do is to remain as patient a possible with your older child, and to offer her as much love and reassurance as you can. Here are a few specific strategies you can use to help your older child feel comfortable with the new baby:

- Set aside a bit of time each day to spend with your older child -- just you and her. Use that time to focus on her, and to do something she enjoys.

- Let her know that her feelings (even feelings of jealously and anger) are natural and understandable. Help her articulate what she's feeling (i.e. "Do you feel angry that mommy is paying attention to the new baby right now, and not to you?"). But remember to explain to your older child that while it's okay to feel her feelings, it's definitely not okay to act on them!

- Offer your older child praise whenever she helps with the new baby, or does something 'nice' for the new baby.

- Help your older child understand that while the new baby has limits, and can't play much yet, there are ways that the new baby can engage. For example, encourage your older child to read a book to the new baby, or to make funny faces at the baby.

- Plan for special activities and outings with grandparents or with you. For example, take her on a run to the store while someone else watches the newborn for half an hour.

- Be sure to set limits with your toddler, and supervise your toddler around the new baby. It's okay to say, "You'll need to wait for a few minutes while I change our baby. Can you get the diaper wipes?" Even a two year old can be a helper and feel happy and useful when they've helped.

There are some great resources out there for preparing toddlers and preschoolers to be big siblings. Two great books, both by Joanna Cole, are *I'm a Big Sister* and *I'm a Big Brother*. Both books are written from the perspective of an older sibling, and both include some nice tips for parents, too! Take heart that even if you have a rough start with the sibling relationship, as with many things, time to adjust makes a big difference!

Safety Tip: Lastly, don't ever leave your toddler unattended with your newborn. Toddlers are unpredictable. It could be something like an emotional outburst of anger or an innocent "helping" of covering the baby with a blanket or feeding him a Cheerio that can be dangerous for the baby

ESSENTIAL KEY #4: ROUTINES AND SLEEP

Approaches to Routines

Routines Can Help Promote Sleep, Especially for Intense Babies

When you create a routine for your baby, you're helping him order his sleep/wake cycles and creating a predictable pattern of events surrounding a certain activity, or set of activities. Routines don't necessarily follow the clock, and they don't have to be rigid; routines can simply be patterns that you and your baby follow to help you both organize your daily and nightly activities. Playing a certain set of lullabies or singing the same song right before bed every day teaches him to associate those activities with sleep. It won't happen right away, but overtime he will learn to associate certain sounds, movements (massage, rocking), and even smells (like lavender, chamomile) with sleep.

The N.A.P.S. Routine: Eat-Sleep-Play

The N.A.P.S. routine is an excellent one for many newborns; it promotes sleep by helping a baby learn to fall asleep on her own. A N.A.P.S. routine works this way:

N - Nurse or Bottle Feed. When your baby wakes from a nap, or at night, offer the breast or bottle.

A - Activity. Follow the feeding with an activity like a diaper change, or a clothing change.

P - Play. Engage your baby in some purposeful interaction, like cuddling, looking at a book, rocking and singing, tummy time, etc.

S - Sleep. After a short period of playtime, put your baby back to bed. Your baby's total awake time, for the feeding, activity time, and playtime, will be about 30-60 minutes in the first month, and about 1 to 2 hours after the first month, for the rest of the newborn stage.

A Sleep-Eat-Sleep Routine

A sleep-eat-sleep routine is perfect for nighttime. At night, you certainly won't want to engage your baby in purposeful activity time after she eats; that will only serve to wake her up! Instead, keep nighttime feedings quiet, and put your baby right back to sleep once she's done feeding.

Sleep-eat-sleep routines are also good for those first few weeks after birth, when your newborn is doing almost nothing but eating and sleeping. It can also be helpful to return to this routine during the growth spurts that happen throughout infancy. Growth spurts may last for 1-3 days. In the newborn stage, growth spurts typically happen at the following times:

- 7-10 days
- 2-3 weeks
- 4-6 weeks
- 3 months

A Sleep-Play-Eat-Sleep Routine

Feeding naturally makes babies sleepy; in the newborn stage, it may be easier on you (and on your newborn) if you have your baby eat right before a nap. This can help your baby fall asleep, and it may make the nap longer and more restful. If you're breastfeeding, nursing will naturally make you and baby sleepy. This can be a good thing, since moms of newborns need naps almost as much as their babies do! Don't worry, the laundry will be there when you wake up. Tip: Try to limit your chores to things you must do (i.e. cook food) to cut back on things that would be nice to do (i.e.

shower — kidding! Showers can be restorative. But, vacuuming the living room can wait one more day, we promise!)

Some parents may be concerned that this kind of routine runs the risk of causing habitual sleep associations (Please see link to additional sleep association article on Resource Page). Although parenting babies to sleep is normal, there are some things you can do to prevent habitual sleep association. You can try to gently teach your baby to go to sleep on her own, instead of being put to sleep by feeding; to do this, feed your baby, then change her diaper, or sing her a special song. This will help gently wake your baby. Then, put her down for her nap, drowsy but at least slightly awake. If you want to help your baby learn to fall asleep on her own, try to put her drown drowsy but slightly awake at bedtime, and for at least two of her naps, as this will help her learn to sleep without being fed to sleep. Remember to listen to your mommy instincts and your baby. If you don't feel your baby is ready for self-soothing and you are happy with your routine, there is no reason to change it.

Asking Friends and Family to Respect Your Baby's Routine

One thing that's challenging, during the newborn stage, is asking those friends and family members who are helping out with the baby to respect your baby's sleep and feeding routines. Well-meaning grandparents or aunts and uncles, who are eager to play with and cuddle your newborn, may inadvertently keep your baby awake well past nap time, or may unintentionally delay a feeding. While this is understandable, do your best to (gently and patiently) remind visitors and helpers that its best for the baby if everyone observes.

It's also a good idea to help your visitors and helpers understand how they can best interact with your newborn. Remind them that newborns become over stimulated quickly, so just being held or spoken to softly is plenty of stimulation for your newborn. Also be aware of how often your newborn is being 'passed around' from one person to another; being passed around can quickly over stimulate and upset a newborn, which will make the next nap or feeding time harder.

Managing Odd Days, Illnesses and Growth Spurts

Routines for Unusual Days

Your newborn is growing rapidly, so you'll need to adapt your routines as your baby changes. You'll also need to alter your routines for those odd days that can crop up - days when your baby is ill, or when your family is traveling, or when your baby is going through a growth spurt.

Routines for Growth Spurts

During a growth spurt, your baby will eat and sleep a lot - in fact, he may do nothing but eat and sleep! And this is normal; during a growth spurt, your baby will need plenty of extra calories. When a growth spurt starts, don't worry about sticking to your normal routine. Instead, take a mini-vacation on your couch. Plan to watch your favorite movies or TV shows, surround yourself with your laptop and phone, stockpile plenty of diapers (for baby) and snacks (for you), and plan to focus on feeding the baby for a few days.

Routines for Travel

Travel can interfere with even the most carefully-planned routines. And that's okay; travel is temporary, and it's wise to plan for the disruptions and inconsistency that travel will cause for you and for your baby, and to be ready to adapt. Feeding times may have to change, and sleeping arrangements may need to be modified.

If you're breastfeeding, nursing covers are great solutions for feeding during travel; they'll help you nurse discreetly. And, if your baby is distractible, a cover can keep him focused on the task at hand. Of course, you may not feel the need to cover up when nursing in public; that's okay. More and more women are choosing to nurse openly. What's more, you may try to cover up, only to find that your baby doesn't like the feel of a wrap covering his body! That's okay, too. To be effective, nursing covers need to work for both you and your baby.

Traveling may disrupt your newborn's regular sleeping patterns and rhythms, especially if your baby will be sleeping in an unfamiliar bed, crib, or bassinet. You can help alleviate your baby's sleeplessness by packing a portable side car or a portable swing (that is, if your newborn likes to sleep in the swing). Portable swings travel well, and they provide an easy way to help soothe a fussy baby to sleep.

If your traveling will involve lots of time spent out and about with your baby, you'll need to plan accordingly, so that naps can happen in the stroller or car seat. Snoozeshade™ makes a variety of products (like car seat covers, stroller covers, and Pack-N-Play™ covers) to help block out the sun and provide a cool, dim environment for baby to nap. Of course, if you're bed-sharing and baby-wearing, you may be able to get by with a firm mattress and the baby wrap or carrier of your choice.

Routines for Illness

As much as it pains us parents to think about it, illness will be a part of your baby's infant and toddler years. While it's important to do what you can to help prevent illness in the newborn stage (since our babies are so fragile in the early weeks and months after birth), sometimes, illness happens despite our best efforts. And, as with growth spurts and travel, illness can wreak havoc on your baby's sleep and feeding routines.

A reminder: it's especially important that you take every precaution you can to prevent illness in the first few weeks after birth. Newborns are especially susceptible to respiratory illnesses; common colds that barely affect children and adults can be potentially deadly for newborns. Babies that are born during cold and flu season (October - April or May, in the United States) may be especially susceptible.

Prevent illness by washing your hands frequently, and requiring anyone who comes into contact with your baby to do the same. Also, keep visitors to a minimum in those early weeks. Most family members and friends will understand if you ask them to postpone their visit until a few weeks after you are home from the hospital.

Often, during an illness, you may notice that your baby wants to sleep more. This is perfectly normal; your newborn's body is working hard to fight off infection, and that's bound to make her a bit sleepier than normal. During her illness, plan to stay home as much as possible, and build in plenty of time for extra sleep.

However, if your newborn is sleeping through feedings, or seems less inclined to eat than normal, you'll want to take him to see a healthcare provider. It's true that your newborn's appetite may decrease a bit during his illness, but if he's skipping feedings entirely or having fewer than normal wet and dirty diapers, he needs medical care.

Many doctors recommend keeping your baby home from public places for the first 6 weeks. This can be difficult for some moms, but it's especially important in the cold months when RSV is a significant danger for newborns. Staying home for the first few weeks allows your baby's immune system to mature, and gives her a much better chance of successfully fighting off an illness later.

Nicole shares:

When my eldest son was just 8-12 weeks old, he contracted RSV and it was so scary hearing his labored breathing all night. We kept him on an incline and kept him close to us and didn't sleep much ourselves for nights while we made sure he was okay. I wouldn't wish that on anyone.

If you're breastfeeding, you may find that your newborn wants to nurse more often than usual. This probably has as much (if not more) to do with comfort as it does with nourishment. If this is the case, let your baby nurse as often as she wants to; it will go a long way towards helping her feel soothed, and it'll ensure that she's getting the nourishment she needs to help her body fight off her illness.

Here's a fun-fact about breastfeeding during your baby's illness: did you know that a breastfeeding mom's body will actually respond to her baby's illness by creating antibodies in the breast milk that are designed to combat the baby's illness? It's true! As little as two hours after a baby has been exposed to a virus, mom's body will begin creating antibodies designed to fight that virus.

Routines for Developmental Transitions

It's hard to see it from day to day, but your newborn is developing at an incredible rate. Your baby is growing bigger and stronger, and his brain is changing rapidly. It makes sense, then, that in the newborn stage, your baby's routines will need to change from month to month (or maybe even week to week).

For example, the sleep and feeding routines that work for your baby during the first month of life will need to change as your baby becomes an older newborn, starting in month two. You may find that your baby is becoming a more efficient feeder, and therefore feeding sessions become shorter. And his sleep may adjust as well: you will likely notice that his awake time starts to get longer and longer, between 1 to 2 hours, and that his sleep starts to sort itself into a handful of longer naps throughout the day (as opposed to 6 or more short cat-naps). Work with your baby to encouraging these longer sleep times. If your newborn has resolved his day/night confusion, you may choose to put him in a quiet and darkened room for his first morning nap and first afternoon nap instead of napping him in a living area. These are usually the first two naps to organize, and although the times will change a bit, these are the naps your baby will rely on through infancy and toddlerhood. The shorter naps are very important at this age, but they usually remain under an hour.

Your baby will have another transition around 3 or 4 months. This will coincide with the 4 month sleep regression (see link on Resources page for additional information on the 4 month sleep regression), a point at which your baby's sleep patterns change significantly (and permanently).

Here's a tip: the growth spurt that happens around 3 months of age is great time to start gently weaning your baby away from her sleep props. Many moms have noticed that growth spurts have two phases – a 1-3 day eating phase followed by a 1-2 day sleeping phase. During the 1-2 days when your baby will be sleeping more than usual you'll have plenty of opportunities to practice weaning away from the sleep props; it also means that the weaning may be a bit easier, since your baby will be extra sleepy and will likely fall asleep faster than she normally would. Just keep in mind that if she's skipping too much sleep with your efforts, it's best to take a break and let her get her rest during a growth spurt.

Helping Your Baby Fall Asleep

In the newborn stage, it's perfectly acceptable for you to help your baby fall asleep when he needs it. As Dr. Sears, author of *The Baby Book*, explains it, newborns need to be "parented" to sleep, instead of being left to fall asleep on their own. With this in mind, you can build some "sleep helps" into your newborn's sleep routines.

Rocking (or Swinging) Your Baby to Sleep

It's no secret that gently rocking a newborn is often a surefire way to put her to sleep. The gentle, repetitive motion that rocking provides mimics the rocking motion that your newborn experienced when she was in the womb; that's probably why newborns find rocking so soothing and relaxing.

This is one reason why infant swings tend to be so effective for so many newborns and young infants (and so popular with their parents!). A swing provides the gentle rocking motion that newborns need to relax and fall asleep, and it provides parents with some much-needed free time, since they don't have to be the ones rocking baby to sleep every few hours. Many infant swings will swing baby back and forth; some, however, provide the option to swing either back-and-forth or side-to-side. Your baby may prefer one type of swinging to another; experiment with different swings (and speeds) to see which your baby prefers.

Swings can also be a great tool for soothing particularly fussy babies.

Nicole remembers using the swing to soothe her oldest son when he was just 6-8 weeks old:

I remember one particularly difficult day when my son was 6-8 weeks old and I could NOT get him to sleep in ANY way whatsoever. Not nursing, holding, cuddling, or swaddling him, or anything. I couldn't take it anymore (he was so fussy) and put him in the swing. He still cried for 10 minutes, but then FINALLY fell asleep! The swing was a Godsend in those early weeks. But, he didn't like 'gentle' swinging. He needed the swing moving fast! Family members teased us we were making him drunk. But, hey, that's what he liked! Later, we learned how to 'hard rock' him in our arms (safely) that mimicked the same movement.

Of course, it may be convenient to let your baby sleep in her swing, but safety must be taken into account, too. The American Academy of Pediatrics released new guidelines in 2011 (3 years after Nicole's son was born) which advised parents to avoid using baby swings as sleep aids. (See link to AAP guidelines on Resource page.) According to the AAP, sitting upright for long periods of time (in a swing, for example, or in a car seat) can make it hard for babies to breathe well, and that can lead to an increased risk of SIDS. Some swings made especially for newborns allow the baby to be in a reclined position that can reduce the risk of the baby's head falling into an unsafe position, so discuss the use of the swing during sleep times with your doctor.

Of course, you don't need a swing to rock your baby; you can do it yourself too! Many cultures around the world encourage rocking babies to sleep at night. Many mothers find this is a very special bonding time with their babies. The time spent holding and touching your baby is very relaxing and healthy for him. Our lives are generally very busy and stopping to rock your baby before bed can give you both the time you need to connect.

Feeding Your Baby to Sleep

As we've already mentioned, sucking is another major reflexive behavior for newborns. The sucking motion is not only necessary for feeding; it's also powerfully comforting and soothing for newborns.

In the early weeks after birth, it may be wise to plan your baby's feedings around her sleep. Plan to nurse before your baby needs a nap; then, your baby will be nice and drowsy when it's time to sleep. In the first few weeks you may use a N.A.P.S. routine for some activity cycles, and use a Sleep-Feed-Sleep routine for other activity cycles depending on the time of day and your baby's needs. As your baby grows, you may be able to use the N.A.P.S. routine throughout the entire day, and then as he leaves the newborn period and his ability to be awake during the day lengthens, you may find he again needs to nurse before and after sleep times. If you would like your baby to go to sleep without your direct intervention you can help by feeding him before sleep but placing him into his sleep space awake. He needs to be aware of the transition between your arms and his bed, so that he isn't surprised when he wakes up in a different place and is not being held by a parent!

Co-Sleeping to Help Your Baby Sleep

Rocking/swinging and sucking are both very soothing to newborns, and incorporating them into your newborn's sleep routines can help greatly in getting your newborn to sleep well. Here's something else that may help your newborn sleep soundly: YOU! That's right; many newborns are soothed and comforted by simply being near mom or dad. Most newborns will sleep well if mom's nearby and can offer a few comforting pats, or a quick nursing, during the night.

Room-Sharing vs. Bed-Sharing

Let's clarify what we mean by "co-sleeping". **Co-sleeping simply means that a child shares a room with a parent.** With that in mind, co-sleeping can mean a baby sleeping in the same bed as his parents; however, it can also mean a baby in a bassinet next to the bed. The American Academy of Pediatrics (AAP) calls that kind of sleeping arrangement "room-sharing".

Room-sharing is considered completely safe, as long as baby's sleeping area follows safety guidelines (no loose bedding, firm mattress that's flush with the sides of the bassinet, tight-fitting bottom sheet, etc.) In fact, the AAP recommends room-sharing as the safest and best sleeping arrangement for infants, especially through the first six months.

Bed-sharing refers to the practice of parents and children sharing the same bed. Some experts (like Dr. James McKenna and Dr. Helen Ball) believe there are ways to bed-share safely, (see link to co-sleeping guidelines on Resource page) but there is a lengthy list of precautions and safety measures that require careful thought and advance planning to implement. For example, it's recommended that you remove pillows and blankets from the bed, and even that you put your mattress directly on the floor. It's also safest if the only people in bed are mom and baby, and baby should sleep beside mom, instead of between mom and dad. In addition, siblings should never share a sleep surface with a baby. What's more, safety guidelines specify that some people should never bed-share, including those who smoke and use drugs/alcohol, those who are extremely obese, and those who are "overly exhausted." That last one is bound to include most parents of newborns! Some research suggests it is particularly dangerous to bed share with newborn babies through the 3rd month, due to their size and inability to move away from dangerous situations.

Dangerous Bed-Sharing Situations

One form of "bed sharing" doesn't involve a bed at all: sometimes, parents sleep with their babies on a couch, or in a recliner. While we understand that it can be so easy to fall asleep with your newborn while relaxing in a recliner, or watching TV on the couch, please understand that this is incredibly dangerous. You should never sleep on a couch or a recliner with your baby. If your baby is hungry and you are sleepy, the floor of a baby proofed area or a firm mattress on the floor is a much safer place to feed him.

Another important reminder: a baby who's swaddled should **never** share a bed with his parents. Remember, when your newborn is swaddled, his movements are restricted; if he's sharing a bed with you, he may be unable to move himself if he ends up in a position that makes it hard for him to breathe.

Bed-Sharing Alternatives

One of the primary reasons parents will bed-share is to enhance the breastfeeding relationship. In the early days after birth, your newborn will wake frequently at night, and will need to feed often. Bed-sharing makes feeding and tending to your newborn simpler and faster, since you have easy access to your baby. It also allows for more skin to skin contact which is very soothing and healthy for babies.

Fortunately, there are alternatives available that provide many of the conveniences of bed-sharing while offering a separate sleeping surface for your baby. One such alternative is the Close and Secure Sleeper™. Nicole used this alternative for a few weeks with her younger son. Designed to fit in an adult bed between mom and dad, the Close and Secure Sleeper™ provides a defined sleeping area for your baby, reducing some of the risks of bed-sharing. Note that this particular co-sleeper is relatively small, making it an option for young infants only. Also, it's designed to fit into a large, king-sized bed.

Another excellent alternative is the Arm's Reach Co-Sleeper™. This co-sleeper offers a separate sleeping area for your newborn, outside of your bed. However, it's designed to fit right up against your bed, with one "wall" of the sleeper dropping down to provide you with easy access to your baby. Miriam shared her bed and used the Arm's Reach Co-Sleeper™ until her babies were able to sit independently.

Our Recommendation: Make informed decisions about sleeping arrangements

Ultimately, decisions about your newborn's sleeping arrangements are best made by you. The Baby Sleep Site® doesn't make recommendations about sleeping surfaces or arrangements, since we realize that every family situation is unique. However, it's our hope that you'll use the information provided in this e-book to make safe, healthy, and informed decisions about your newborn's sleeping conditions. If you have further questions about the best sleeping arrangements for your newborn, we recommend that you speak with your baby's healthcare provider or your lactation consultant.

Helping Baby to Sleep vs. Letting Baby Fall Asleep Independently

In the early days and weeks after your baby is born, you'll probably find that you're putting your baby to sleep quite often -- by nursing, feeding, rocking, or holding him until he finally drifts off to sleep. This is perfectly fine during the newborn period, so if you find that putting your baby to sleep has become a regular part of his sleep routine, don't worry about it. Babies this age may need help navigating the transition between sleep and wake states. Remember, your newborn is far too young to cry in a manipulative way, or in an effort to "make" you do something.

When it's possible, try to create a situation in which your newborn is able to fall asleep, independently. This doesn't mean laying him down wide awake and screaming, of course! Rather, try to lay your newborn down for sleep when she's drowsy and calm, but slightly awake. Or, if your baby falls asleep during a feeding, try to rouse her slightly by changing her diaper, or singing to her, or even changing her position in your arms. Then, when she's a bit awakened, lay her down to sleep.

If parent-dependent sleep props become a problem as your baby gets a bit older, you'll begin to wean him off rocking or feeding to sleep, and help him gradually learn to fall asleep on his own, without any help from you. This will help him learn to sleep better at night, and to take long, restorative naps. Don't stress about needing to put your baby to sleep. That's a perfectly normal and appropriate thing to do in the newborn stage and can work for some babies throughout infancy and into toddlerhood.

Some parents observe that their babies only sleep when being held. If you think about it, when you have a newborn, just a few weeks ago they were being "held" 24/7 in the womb, so it's not unreasonable for them to need a LOT of holding and cuddling the first weeks and months. We encourage you to embrace your role as a baby holder and carrier! However, we do encourage parents to put their babies down a few times per day for a few minutes each time beginning as early as the first few days. We don't necessarily expect your baby to sleep, but this will help them become accustomed to the sensation of lying flat instead of being all curled up; it's kind of like baby yoga, since they'll be all stretched out for the first time! Babies need Stretch Time just like they need Tummy Time during the day. Stretch Time happens with mom's arms curled around the baby while they lay on the floor or even on a firm mattress. If you feel that your baby won't sleep without being held try this: feed your baby; make sure he has a clean diaper, then use the 5 "s" we reviewed earlier and place him in a swing with a swaddle and pacifier, while you grab a shower or a snack. Then once you get him up, spend some time skin to skin or put him in a safe wrap or baby carrier for extra bonding.

Developing Healthy Sleep Habits

In the early weeks after birth, don't spend too much time worrying about your baby's sleeping patterns (or lack of sleeping patterns, as it may be!) Instead, focus on enjoying your little one and getting as much sleep as you can yourself. This is what you can expect during the newborn period:

Birth – 8 weeks: Get your baby to sleep anyway you can. Focus on enjoying your new baby and getting to know each other. If independent sleep is important to you, begin now by allowing him to fall to sleep independently for two naps and bedtime. All naps may take place in a living area to help resolve day/night confusion. Keep in mind that these efforts should be consistent, yet very gentle and distress- free for mom and baby. And don't worry if your efforts don't work right way; some newborns need to be soothed to sleep for all sleep times.

8 weeks – 12 weeks: At this age we expect day/night confusion to be resolved. Your baby may go ONE 4-6 hour stretch between feedings at night, but otherwise needs to feed every 2-3 hours for breast fed babies and 3-4 hours for formula fed babies around the clock. Continue to put your baby down for his first morning nap and first afternoon nap. These naps should take place in a quiet, darkened room.

12 weeks- 16 weeks: Continue putting your baby down awake at bedtime and for two of his naps. Some babies this age will have one 5-8 hour stretch of sleep. Others will still only have a 4-6 hour stretch. If you are feeling overwhelmed by a lack of sleep and your baby doesn't have a longer sleep stretch that coincides with your sleep, at least four to six hours in length, the Baby Sleep Site® may be able to help with a Personalized Sleep Plan™.

16 weeks and beyond: Identify your baby's sleep associations, and begin to slowly and gently wean her away from them. Is there something your baby needs in order to fall asleep? Does she need to suck on her pacifier? Does she need you to rock her or feed her to sleep? All of these are sleep associations - things your baby needs in order to fall asleep. If you notice that your baby is waking every 1-2 hours during the night and can't get back to sleep without her sleep prop, it may be time to gently work toward breaking the habit. We always feed a hungry baby and comfort a lonely or frightened baby, but there are gentle things we can do to encourage the kind of self-soothing that helps babies navigate within and between sleep cycles.

Once your baby is gaining weight well, begin gently establishing healthy sleep routines and schedules. Don't focus on a by-the-clock schedule at this age; instead, encourage any natural sleep and feeding patterns your baby may develop, and begin working towards a predictable and consistent schedule. This won't happen right away, but you can start moving in this direction once your baby is a few months old.

Begin as you mean to continue. Once your baby is 8-12 weeks old, evaluate his current sleep routines. Is he regularly napping in his swing? Do you have to nurse him to sleep after every nighttime waking? If these are things you would like to change, gently begin steering your baby towards sleeping arrangements and routines that will work better for everyone. It's much easier to help a 2 month old to fall asleep without parent-dependent sleep props at some sleep times than it is a 9 month old who is used to being fed and rocked to sleep for all naps, bedtime, and any night waking.

Stay consistent. It can be easy to try a technique for a few days, only to become frustrated and give up. But it's important that you remain consistent as you set the stage for sleep, even if you work only on bedtime or two naps per day. Don't feel like you need to work on sleep coaching all day long. Try out a new sleep coaching technique for at least 1-2 weeks (unless you or baby feel distressed); it may take that long for you to see any results.

Depending on your baby's temperament, sleep coaching at a young age can be easy or hard, just like any age. But keep in mind that it's never too early to begin gently sleep coaching - especially if you know your family needs it. One particular family we worked with had an 8 week old at home who wasn't sleeping well at all. The mom's sleep was so disrupted, and she became so exhausted, that she ended up with postpartum depression. At this point, the whole family was suffering; they had trouble coping with even ordinary, day-to-day struggles. Fortunately, they knew that in cases like this, it's best to be proactive. They contacted us, and we began sleep coaching.

It went much better than any of us could have anticipated! We started with the Fading Method, and encouraged the baby to learn to fall asleep from a drowsy state, without the pacifier and without help from mom. Mom stayed by the baby the entire time, patting and shushing him for comfort when necessary. There were times she had to pick him up to calm him down, and every day wasn't perfect, but after our work together, the family was able to function again. This is such a good reminder that it's never too early to start helping your newborn learn healthy sleeping habits.

CONCLUSION

By now, you might be feeling like a bit of an expert in newborn sleep. And you should! After reading this book, you likely have a much better understanding of the 4 keys to your newborn's sleep:

Your newborn's **feeding** is closely connected with his sleep. In fact, his feeding needs will drive his sleep patterns.

Your newborn's methods of **communicating** (vocalizations, reflexive cues, and body language) reveal a lot about his feeding and sleep needs. Once you learn to "decode" his language, it'll help you better meet and even anticipate his needs.

Your newborn can benefit from a simple **schedule** in the first few months after birth, since it will help her sort out her days and nights.

Flexible, predictable **routines** associated with feeding and sleep can go a long way towards soothing fussy and intense newborns and can help promote longer, better sleep.

The road to a good night's sleep won't always be easy and smooth; there are bound to be some bumps along the way! But knowing and understanding the 4 keys to newborn sleep will help you and your baby achieve healthy sleep habits that will last a lifetime. We hope these keys will help you on your journey, and most of all that you'll make incredible memories and have special times with your newborn!

ABOUT THE AUTHORS

Nicole Johnson

My name is Nicole Johnson and I am a married mother of two wonderful boys, as well as the Senior Baby Sleep Consultant and owner of The Baby Sleep Site®.

When my eldest son was a baby, he had a lot of sleep problems. Sleep like a baby? Yeah, right! You had better hope you never sleep like my baby did. He would wake up every one or two hours, ALL NIGHT LONG. I had to do so much to get him through the night.

By thoroughly researching the key literature and scientific reports, I became an expert in sleep methods, scheduling routines, baby and toddler development needs and more. I overcame my son's sleeping issues in a way that matched my own parenting style, and knew it was my mission to help other tired parents "find their child's sleep."

I started by leading an Internet-based message board and helped countless parents just like you overcome their own sleeping challenges much quicker and faster than I had. I then created my website in 2008 and expanded my offerings to include e-books, articles, a blog, and customized sleep consulting. The feedback around the world has been incredible!

I would love to help you with your challenge. Know that I never offer one-size-fits-all advice or pass judgment on your parenting philosophies. I incorporate who you are and what your child is undergoing to create a unique service. And I will give you the support you need to see your challenge through to the end.

Miriam Chickering

Miriam Chickering is the mother to five children, a writer, editor, and consultant. She is a Registered Nurse with a Bachelors of Science in Nursing and a Board Certified Lactation Consultant (IBCLC.) Her other work includes *The Gentle Art of Mothering*, a faith-based book about newborn care. As an educator, Miriam loves teaching nursing students in the clinical setting and working with new families during prenatal classes, home visits, and hospital stays. As a sleep consultant with The Baby Sleep Site® Miriam enjoys helping all mothers achieve healthy sleep for themselves and their babies, and specializes in balancing sleep needs with a good breastfeeding relationship.

ABOUT THE BABY SLEEP SITE®

The Baby Sleep Site® (http://www.babysleepsite.com) specializes in baby sleep products and consulting services. The company was founded by Nicole Johnson, sleep coach, wife, and the mother of two boys. Nicole received an honorary degree in "Surviving Sleep Deprivation," thanks to her son's "no sleep" curriculum. She became an expert on infant and toddler sleep and made it her mission to help other parents solve their child's sleep problems, too. All sleep consultants are carefully chosen by Nicole, with their diverse backgrounds in mind. They go through extensive training to learn the strategies and philosophies of The Baby Sleep Site® in order to provide you with a knowledgeable, thoughtful, supportive, and consistent experience no matter where you are in your journey to better sleep.

Over 500,000 parents visit The Baby Sleep Site® website each month to find solutions for their children's sleep problems, including personalized, one-on-one sleep consultations, comprehensive e-books on sleeping through the night, schedules and taking better naps, free articles and blogs on timely topics, and strong community.

Whether a family is struggling with a baby who won't fall asleep at night or a toddler who just doesn't want to nap, The Baby Sleep Site® tailors every approach with individuality in mind. We never offer one-size-fits-all advice or pass judgment on individual parenting philosophies.

If you have any questions or comments on this guide, please e-mail contact@babysleepsite.com.

While The Baby Sleep Site® publishes what we consider to be safe tips and suggestions, all The Baby Sleep Site® content is made available on an as-is basis, with no warrantees expressed or implied. As such, readers use any advice at their own risk.

ADDITIONAL SUPPORT AND RESOURCES

Resource Page

Please visit the Resource page online for links to articles, videos and websites mentioned throughout the book:

http://www.babysleepsite.com/essential-keys-resource-links

Additional Support

This book is designed to provide you with the tools and strategies you need to help your baby establish healthy feeding and sleep habits during the newborn stage. However, as your baby grows, you may find that you need additional sleep help and support. With that in mind, we invite you to take to take advantage of these <u>free</u> Baby Sleep Site® resources:

- For babies 3 months or older, you can download a copy of our free guide on night sleep: ***5 Ways To Help Your Child Sleep Through The Night*** (http://www.babysleepsite.com/baby-sleep-through-night-free-ebook/). This straightforward, easy-to-read e-Book is packed with useful information that you can put to work right away - including gentle, tear-free ways to help your baby learn to fall asleep independently and sleep through the night.

- Naps are problematic for lots of families. If your baby is struggling to take long, restorative naps, and if you are having a hard time establishing a consistent daily nap schedule, download a copy of our free nap guide: *7 **Common Nap Mistakes*** (http://www.babysleepsite.com/free-baby-nap-guide/). This e-Book lays out common nap mistakes that families make, and offers tried-and-true steps parents can take to help their babies get the nap time rest they need to be healthy.

- Sleep problems do not disappear when babies are older (unfortunately!) Plenty of toddlers continue to wake often at night, and to resist naps. As your baby grows into a toddler, if you continue to struggle with sleep, why not download a copy of our free guide on toddler sleep: ***Toddler Sleep Secrets*** (http://www.babysleepsite.com/toddler-sleep-training-secrets-free-ebook/). This free e-Book highlights proven methods that are designed to help your toddler sleep through the night and take longer, more restful naps.

The Baby Sleep Site® also offers a variety of paid resources, designed to help tired families get the rest they need:

- You can purchase a copy of one of our **comprehensive e-Books** on newborn, baby, toddler, and nap sleep by visiting our Products page (http://www.babysleepsite.com/baby-sleep-products/).

- You can join our **Members Area**, and receive access to all of our sleep e-Books (as well as case studies, tele-seminars, and weekly member chats) by visiting our Membership page (http://www.babysleepsite.com/become-a-member/).

- You can receive personal, one-on-one help from a highly-trained sleep consultant by purchasing one of our **consultation packages** (https://www.babysleepsite.com/baby-toddler-sleep-consulting-services/). Your consultation will include a Personalized Sleep Plan™, written especially for your family and tailored to your baby's unique temperament and needs.

Be sure to check out these additional free resource and helps, too:

- Consider reading our **Baby Sleep Site® blog** at http://www.babysleepsite.com/blog, updated twice a week with helpful, sleep-focused articles.

- Like us on **Facebook** (http://facebook.com/babysleepsite), and join other tired parents on the journey to better sleep!

- Read our **parent stories** (http://www.babysleepsite.com/testimonials/) and see what kind of difference The Baby Sleep Site® has made (and continues to make) in the lives of families around the world.

Ordering Additional Copies

If you would like to order additional copies of this booklet, please visit us at:

http://babysleepsite.com/essential-keys-ordering

Made in the USA
San Bernardino, CA
22 November 2013